CHAIR YOGA FOR SENIORS

CONTENTS

BALANCE EXERCISES
FOR SENIORS

CONTENTS

WALL PILATES FOR SENIORS

CONTENTS

CHAIR YOGA FOR SENIORS

STRETCHES FOR PAIN RELIEF AND JOINT HEALTH
THAT IMPROVE SENIORS' FLEXIBILITY TO HELP
PREVENT FALLS AND IMPROVE QUALITY OF LIFE

FIT FOREVER

INTRODUCTION

Yoga is an ancient practice that has its roots in Eastern Asian tradition. It combines breathing, movement, and meditation to promote emotional, mental, and physical wellness. In the last few decades, yoga has become an increasingly popular form of exercise, particularly in the West. There are indeed many types and forms of yoga, but they are all designed to encourage overall health and wellness.

For many, traditional yoga can seem a bit overwhelming, especially for those of us who are no longer as steady on our feet as we once were or even for those of us who just feel better sitting. This is where chair yoga comes in!

Chair yoga offers all the benefits of traditional yoga but with the security of a chair to keep you firmly grounded. Like traditional yoga, chair yoga can help with pain and stress relief, and it can also assist with joint lubrication, balance, and the effects of arthritis.

This book has been specifically designed with seniors in mind who would like to begin or continue a yoga practice. It includes step-by-step guides for the various poses as well as variations depending on your comfort level. There are beginner, intermediate, and advanced chair poses that can be practiced as individual sequences or that can be combined to create a unique sequence that works for you.

Now that you've made the decision to add more movement to your daily routine, it is important that you consult with your doctor before you begin. Take the time to discuss your specific needs and how best to start your yoga practice. Not everyone will begin at the same level or progress in the same way. Once you've got the green light, remember to take it slow and do what feels right for you. Above all, have fun.

GETTING STARTED WITH CHAIR YOGA

As we age, our muscle strength declines affecting our legs, hips, and core. Chair yoga can help us to restore and maintain our spine health. Poor posture and weak spinal muscles can affect all parts of our bodies so having a regular chair yoga practice can help reverse or slow down some of the effects of aging on our bodies.

PSYCHOLOGICAL BENEFITS

Yoga connects the body to the mind and the mind to the spirit through the breath and helps us to be fully present in the moment and be aware. It can positively affect our mood as well as our cognitive function and can provide us with a sense of well-being and satisfaction.

Many seniors suffer from anxiety and worry, particularly about losing their independence or self-sufficiency. The focus on breathing and the breath in yoga can aid in soothing the mind and body and reducing the body's stress response. When practiced regularly, in a tranquil environment, it can alleviate stress and help bring peace and calm. We will explore the benefits of the breath in an upcoming chapter to better understand how breathing can impact the body and mood.

As with our physical bodies as we age, the structure and function of our brain change and decline. This can lead to impaired memory or reduced attention. Yoga can help stop the decline of brain function. In yoga, the brain has to focus and concentrate on performing the yoga poses or on meditating. This training of the brain to focus increases or improves attention, awareness, and memory (Hastings, 2017).

PHYSICAL BENEFITS

We have already established that physical activity, particularly for seniors, helps with mobility and strength as well as weight management and heart health. Yoga can improve balance, strength, and stability and can even slow down or reverse the loss of all of those. Just 20 minutes a day can improve your overall health and strength.

According to the Centers for Disease Control, falling is one of the main causes of injury and death among persons over 65 (Lehmkuhl, 2020). Being physically active and strengthening the muscles of your legs, hips, and core can go a long way in preventing falls and increasing your mobility. The more movement you can incorporate into your daily routine the better your balance will be. This means that you will be better able to perform your daily tasks. Staying physically active as you age can ensure that you maintain your independence.

As we age, our bones also become brittle, which means it is easier to break a bone if you fall. Doing yoga can help to strengthen your bones and delay or prevent the onset of osteoporosis. Yoga can, in fact, increase your bone density even as you get older.

Yoga can also increase your stamina and control joint inflammation and pain associated with many chronic conditions. This means that you can have the confidence to live and move independently.

The regular practice of yoga reduces your chance of having heart disease and of becoming a Type 2 diabetic. It also lowers your blood pressure and can alleviate aches and pains associated with aging. Importantly, it helps you to breathe better. Many people have difficulty breathing as they get older and a lack of oxygen to the cells can have detrimental effects on your body. Yoga teaches you how to focus on your breathing to maximize the flow of oxygen.

Yoga, or chair yoga in our case, can have a positive impact on our overall health—psychologically, emotionally, and physically. You can practice chair yoga anywhere, anytime in small groups or by yourself. You really don't need a lot to do it and the outcomes you gain by just doing 20 minutes a day are tremendous.

WHAT YOU NEED

As with any physical activity, it is always important to check with your doctor or healthcare professional before beginning. Chair yoga is a gentle form of exercise that does not have a lot of impact on the joints or muscles but it is still advisable to get the okay from your medical adviser.

For chair yoga, all you need is a non-cushioned chair with a straight back and no arms and, if possible, a set of two-pound hand weights and a yoga block. You should wear loose, comfortable clothing that is easy to move in and won't be restrictive. It is better to practice your yoga barefooted. If you're practicing on tiles or hardwood floors try to avoid socks because they may be slippery.

Find a space that works for you and that you will enjoy returning to on a daily basis. Make sure that the space you choose is big enough for your chair and you to fully extend your arms and legs. When choosing or creating your space, let it reflect your personality or what you want to feel in that space but don't let it be cluttered. Clutter will distract you from your practice. Remember the goal of your space should be to keep you calm, focused, and at peace.

Once you've found your space, the next step is to choose the time of day that works best for you. In the beginning, you may want to try doing your practice at different times and notice how you feel or if there are any distractions. Whatever time you choose, try to be consistent. It helps you to create a routine for your body and mind.

If you have never tried yoga before then it is probably best to start with the beginner poses and then work your way up as you get stronger and more confident. If you've been physically active you can opt for the intermediate poses but still check with your doctor first. Also, ensure that you are hydrated before and after your practice. Most importantly, relax and have fun.

2

BREATHING IN YOGA

Any yoga practice begins and ends with the breath. Breathing or *pranayama,* as it is called in yoga, is the quintessential feature of yoga. It is considered to be the *vital energy*. Awareness of your breath and matching your breathing to your movement is what defines yoga and makes it a whole-body experience as opposed to just an exercise.

When we become aware of our breath and our breathing, our mind becomes quieter, stiller. As a result, we become calmer and less agitated. Our breathing sends signals to our brain that, in turn, cause our bodies to react in certain ways. Breathing deeply and slowly tells our brain that everything is okay and that it is safe to relax and be at peace.

As we breathe deeply, the *vital energy* starts to push through our emotional and physical blockages and stresses. This movement of the *vital energy* throughout our body is what gives us the "feel good" sensation we experience at the end of our practice. In general, our heart beats more slowly when we exhale. Yoga uses breathing techniques to work with our body's natural responses to create that calming effect.

It is important to note though that *pranayama* is not rigorous breath control that results in discomfort or harm. It is also not an exercise; it is an awareness that can help to balance the physical, mental, and subtle bodies.

THE BREATH AND ITS BENEFITS

We've been breathing all our lives so we shouldn't need to be taught how to breathe, right? For the most part, this is true. Yoga is not about teaching you how to breathe properly; it's about helping you to become more aware of your breath and how it changes depending on what you're doing or how you're feeling. The notion of *pranayama* is to marry the breath to your activities, whether it's during your practice or your daily life. It is about paying attention and focusing on yourself—emotionally, mentally, and physically.

It is best to breathe in and out through your nose. Your nose is your body's natural air filter and can warm or cool the air as needed. The nose protects you against millions of foreign particles that circulate in the air. Moreover, breathing through your nose can reduce the rate of exertion during exercise or daily activities, which means that you will feel less tired during and after activity if you breathe through your nose. Furthermore, because the way we breathe sends signals to our brain, taking breaths through your nose reduces your nervous system's "fight or flight" response to situations.

Deep breathing and an awareness of your breath can lower your cortisol levels, the hormones responsible for stress. More importantly, it can help reduce your feelings of anxiety and depression. Focus on your breath can stabilize and even lower your blood pressure levels as well as strengthen your core. It can also counteract insomnia and sleeplessness. Overall, *pranayama* positively impacts your physical, emotional, and mental well-being.

BREATHING TECHNIQUES

Simple Breath

This technique is particularly beneficial for grounding and comfort and is the basis of many other breathing techniques.

1. Breathe in and out through your nose.
2. Begin to notice your breath without altering it.
3. Once you're comfortable, start to pay attention to the rhythm of your inhale and exhale.
4. Over time, begin to notice the space between your inhale and exhale as well as the pause between the two.
5. Continue as needed.

Yogic Breath

This technique helps to manage and ease anxiety and gives you that "feel good" sensation.

1. Begin with the simple breath technique.
2. When you're comfortable, begin to pay attention to the flow of air into the belly button towards the pubic bone as you breathe in and out and as the belly deflates as you breathe out.

3. Next, pay attention to how your rib cage expands as your belly button rises on your inhale and how your rib cage contracts and your belly deflates as you breathe out.
4. Allow yourself to become relaxed as your body embraces your breath.
5. Continue as needed until you are ready to complete your breathing practice.

Golden Thread Breath

If you suffer from insomnia or any kind of pain, this technique will provide the comfort and relief you need.

1. Start by establishing your yogic breath.
2. Once you are comfortable, begin to relax the muscles of your jaw and throat, and unclench your teeth. Create a small space between your teeth as well as your lips.
3. Keeping the breath gentle and steady, inhale through the nose and exhale through the tiny space between the lips.
4. Begin to focus on your exhale, and if possible, try to lengthen it slightly.
5. Continue this technique as desired, until you are ready to complete your practice.

Pranayama can benefit anyone and can be done anywhere. There is no special equipment or time frame. You simply take a few moments to bring awareness to your breath in any or all of your daily activities. Many times in yoga though, *pranayama* is part of a broader meditation practice. We will briefly explore meditation in the next chapter before moving on to the chair yoga poses.

3

MEDITATION

Meditation has been practiced by many different cultures worldwide for centuries. In its literal sense, meditation means to reflect upon or contemplate. In yoga, meditation relates to the awareness of the interconnectedness of all living things. It is more than simply concentration; it is a widening of your state of awareness. The first step in meditation is stilling the mind. This in turn relaxes your nervous system and allows you to focus and become aware of things around you.

Chair yoga is great because the poses in this form of yoga can be meditative in and of themselves. *Pranayama* and the yoga poses combined help to prepare your body for meditation by encouraging us to focus on our posture and our breathing. Additionally, like chair yoga itself, meditation can be practiced anywhere, at any time.

IMPORTANCE AND BENEFITS OF MEDITATION

We often rush through our days and our routines, not paying attention to the steps and details that led us through these moments. We tend to be disconnected from our present, many times because we are focused on what is supposed to happen next or worrying about what came before.

Meditation helps to center and ground us and make us more mindful, not only of our surroundings but of our actions and thoughts. It can create feelings of peace and ease and can help to release your body of unwanted tension. Through meditation and the expansion of your awareness, you give your active mind a chance to rest and release the constant thoughts and stressors.

In effect, a regular meditation practice can act as a form of stress management and aid in increasing your emotional well-being. It may also aid in managing your symptoms of anxiety, depression, sleeplessness, and pain. Meditation also improves your memory and can boost your immunity.

Combining *pranayama* with your meditation practice is beneficial to your overall health and wellness. It will leave you feeling alert and refreshed. Meditation is a great way to begin or end your day or to help you deal with any difficulties that may arise during the course of your day.

PRACTICING CHAIR MEDITATION

Before you embark on a meditation practice, it is important for you to remember to be patient and kind to yourself. Meditation takes time so start slowly, for short periods of time. Don't expect to be able to meditate for 30 minutes on your first try. It is a practice because you have to train your mind and body to relax and be receptive.

Like your yoga practice, you also need to set a schedule for your meditation practice. Again, find the time of day that works best for you and has the least amount of disruptions or interruptions. It may be easiest to practice your meditation at the end of your yoga chair practice. Create a space that is comfortable and welcoming and free from clutter.

Most importantly, be comfortable. If you are fidgeting or in any distress, you will not gain the benefits of your practice. There is no one posture for meditation. Select the way that you can sustain for the length of your practice and again, choose clothing that is loose and easy to move in.

Chair Meditation

1. Sit up tall in your chair and place your feet flat on the floor, hip-distance apart. Slouching will constrict your breathing.
2. Ground down through your sitz bones (bottom part of your pelvis) and relax your shoulders back and down, away from your ears.
3. If it feels comfortable, close your eyes or gently lower and soften your gaze. Rest your hands on your thighs with your palms facing up. This gesture creates openness and receptivity.
4. Begin to notice your breath and perhaps practice one of the breathing techniques.
5. To come out of your meditation, begin to return to your normal breathing, then gently open your eyes. Give yourself a moment to assimilate the sensations.

BEGINNER POSES

If you're just getting started with a physical fitness routine or you're new to yoga then this is a great place to start. The yoga poses in this section are meant to provide you with a firm foundation. They are the poses you can use as you build your practice and you will be able to add more to them as you move along.

The poses highlighted here can be done in sequence to provide you with a 20-minute practice. If you include *pranayama* and meditation at the end of the sequence you will have about a 30-minute practice. Most importantly, take your time and enjoy each moment of your practice.

MOUNTAIN POSE

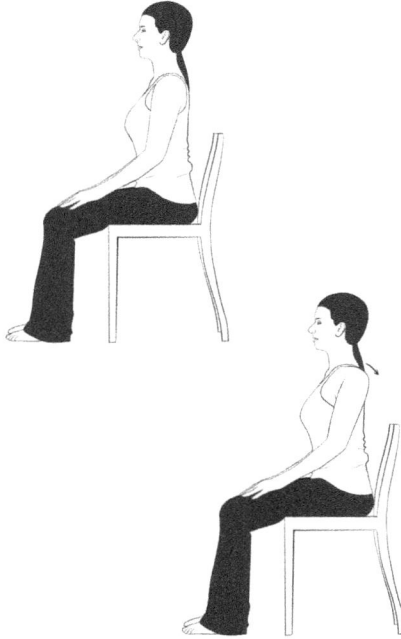

This is a great pose to begin your practice. It engages your core muscles as you sit up tall and helps you focus on your breath and check in with your posture. You can return to this pose after each pose in the sequence.

To begin:

1. Take a deep inhale and sit up tall in your chair, extending your spine.
2. Keep your feet flat on the floor with your knees hip-width apart and your toes pointing forward. Rest your hands, palms facing up, gently on your thighs.
3. Take another deep breath in and as you exhale, gently roll your shoulders back and away from your ears.
4. Engage your core as you become heavy on your sitting bones and lengthen through your spine. Keep your feet firmly pressed into the ground.

SIDE NECK STRETCHES

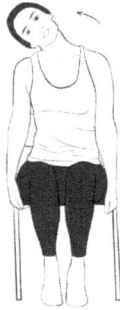

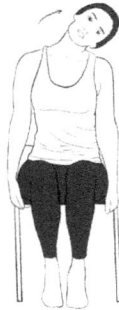

These stretches are a great way to reduce tension in the neck and shoulders and help you to relax your jaw and facial muscles.

1. Begin in Mountain pose.
2. Sit up tall as you inhale.

3. As you exhale, slowly drop your right ear to your right shoulder. Notice if your shoulders are tense and reaching towards your ear. Try to relax your shoulders and roll them back and down.

4. Inhale and lift your head back up to a neutral position.

5. Now, exhale again and drop your left ear to your left shoulder. Again, observe your shoulders and try to keep them relaxed and down, away from the ears.

6. Inhale and return your head to its neutral position.

7. Try to do this pose at least 3 times on each side. You can do more if it feels good and you feel that your body needs it.

SHOULDER ROLLS

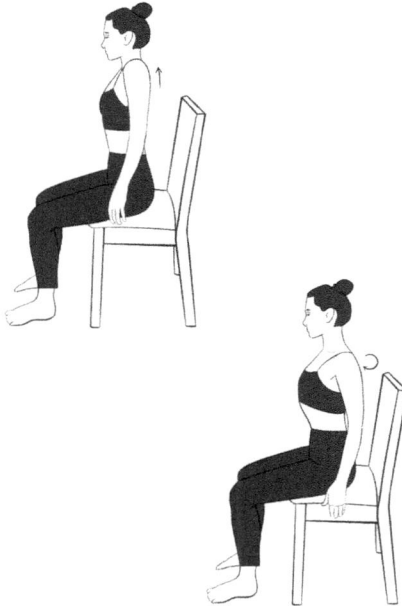

Shoulder rolls help to open up the shoulders and improve mobility in the shoulder joints. This ensures that you can easily and confidently complete daily tasks.

1. Begin by sitting in Mountain pose.
2. Inhale and lift your shoulders up, then back. As you exhale, bring your shoulders down and around back to your starting position. You should make a full circle with your shoulders with each cycle of breath.
3. Try to keep the movement of your shoulders smooth and continuous.
4. After five circles like this, reverse the movement bringing your shoulders up and forward as you inhale and down and around as you return to the start. This direction may feel a bit strange but that's how it should be. Complete five circles in this direction.

VOLCANO ARMS

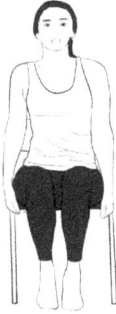

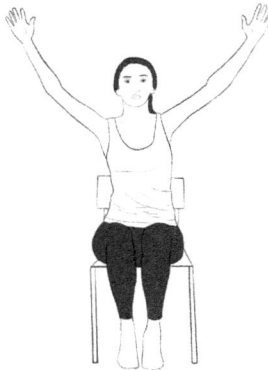

This pose gently stretches your shoulders, arms, and chest and can help improve your mobility in the shoulder joints.

1. Start in Mountain pose.
2. As you inhale, slowly begin to lift both arms above your head in the shape of a V. Notice if

your shoulders are lifting up towards your ears and try to relax your shoulders down.

3. As you exhale, lower your arms to the starting position.
4. Repeat this pose at least 3 more times and try to match your breathing to your movements. If it feels uncomfortable to lift your arms all the way up, just go as far as feels good and doesn't cause any discomfort.

SEATED ONE-LEGGED MOUNTAIN

This pose engages your core muscles, which are critical for sitting, standing, walking, and movement in general. It also helps to tone and strengthen your quadriceps.

1. Begin in Mountain pose, sitting up tall with your shoulders relaxed away from your ears and your feet firmly on the floor with your legs at right angles.
2. Inhale and slowly lift your right knee up and then lower it. Only lift your knee as high as feels good to you. You should not feel any pain or discomfort. Lower your foot as you exhale.
3. Repeat this ten times with each leg, then return to the Mountain pose and observe your breath.

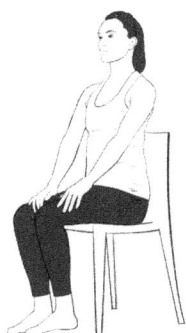

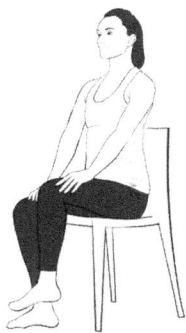

KNEE SWINGS

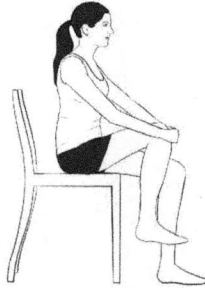

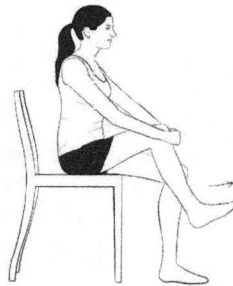

Knee swings are a good way to strengthen the muscles around your knees. They also help to increase the range of motion and mobility in your knees. Strong knee muscles and joints can protect you from knee injuries as you age.

1. Begin in Mountain pose with your belly button pulled in and your shoulders relaxed away from your ears.
2. If you can, clasp your hand under your right knee and begin to kick your right leg back and forth. If reaching under your knee is difficult, you can sit back in your chair and kick your right leg back and forth.
3. Repeat these steps for your left leg. Remember, only lift your leg as high as feels comfortable and go at a pace that is sustainable for you. Also, make sure you note your breath.
4. Try to do at least 10 swings on each side.

LEG LIFTS WITH POINT AND FLEX

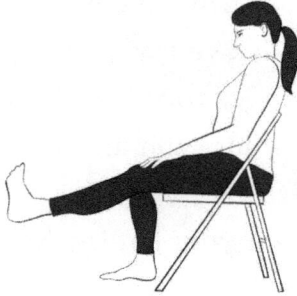

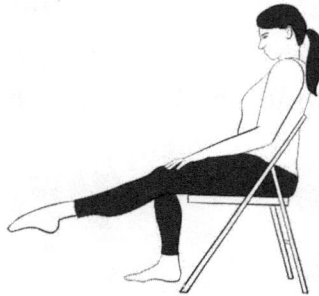

Leg lifts are good for toning your quadriceps and engaging your core. Pointing and flexing your feet help to stretch the muscles in your shin and calf and increases mobility in the foot.

1. Start by sitting up tall in your chair with your feet firmly touching the ground and your hands resting anywhere that is comfortable.
2. As you breathe in, extend your right leg out in front of you. Only go as high or as far as feels good for you. With your leg extended, point and flex your right foot a few times. This can be done quickly or slowly depending on how you feel.
3. On an exhale, slowly lower your right foot.
4. Repeat the movement with your left leg and foot and try to do at least five on each side. As you get stronger and more confident you can increase the number of lifts.

FULL BODY STRETCH

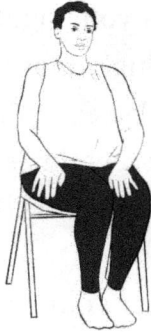

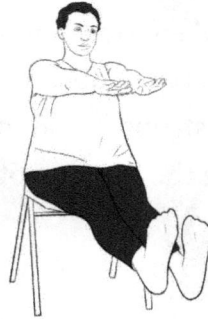

This pose engages all the muscles in your body and helps to strengthen them. It is also a great way to end your practice.

1. Begin in Mountain pose with your knees hip-width apart and your core engaged.

2. As you inhale, slowly and gently lift your arms and legs up at the same time. Try not to slouch as you do this. Only lift as far as you can.
3. On an exhale, return to the Mountain pose. Repeat this movement at least three times.
4. When you return to the Mountain pose after your last stretch, take a few minutes to relax and observe your breath and the sensations in your body.

5

INTERMEDIATE POSES

As you get stronger or if you are physically active then you may consider trying these poses. You can add them to the Beginner poses for a longer, more fluid practice or you can do them on their own. No matter what you decide, you will benefit from this practice. For these poses, you can add a set of two-pound weights. As always, check with your doctor before you begin, be sure to stay hydrated, and have fun.

SHOULDER ROLLS WITH HANDS

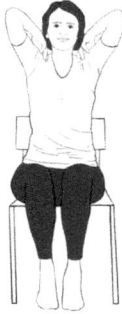

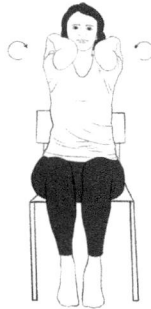

This movement is great for warming up your upper back and shoulders and releasing any tension. It also increases mobility in the shoulder joints.

1. Begin in Mountain pose and place your fingertips on your shoulders.

2. Begin to make circles with your shoulders, using your elbows to guide you. Go as slow or as fast as feels comfortable and be sure to notice your breath as you do your circles.

3. After five complete circles in one direction, reverse your circles and do five more.

WARRIOR II ARMS WITH FISTS

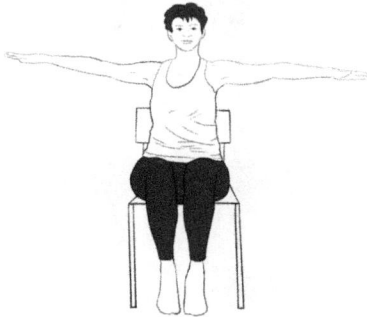

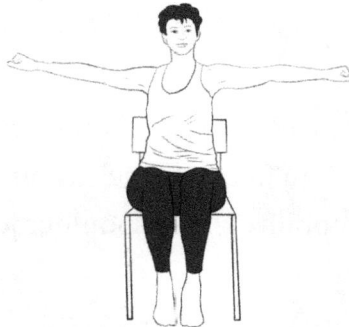

This pose engages the muscles of your upper arms and shoulders and strengthens your hands and fingers. It is especially beneficial to those suffering from carpal tunnel syndrome.

1. Start in Mountain pose, making sure that your feet are firmly planted on the ground and that you are sitting up straight. Remember, slouching will diminish your breathing and make the pose more difficult.
2. Slowly extend both arms up and out to your sides until they are shoulder level. Don't worry if you can't quite reach there yet, just go as far as you can.
3. Keeping your arms lifted, inhale and squeeze your fingers into tight fists. As you exhale, stretch the fingers as wide as you can, exaggerating the movement. Lower the arms.
4. Repeat this movement at least eight more times.

SEATED SIDE TWIST

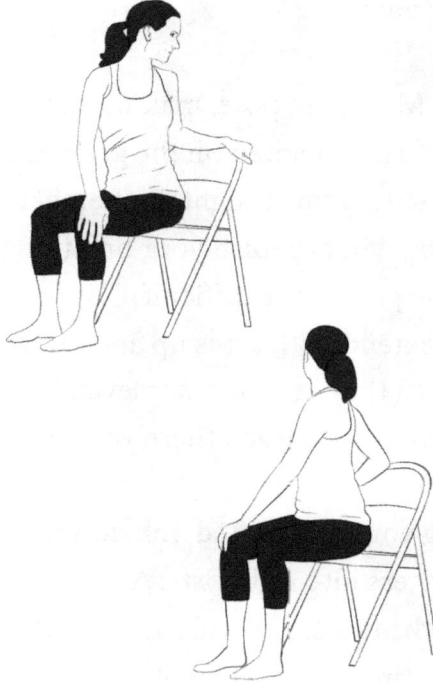

The movements involved in this pose help to tone your waistline while engaging your core. It also increases flexibility in your spine.

1. Again, begin in Mountain pose keeping a nice straight back with your shoulders down and away from your ears.
2. Inhale and gently twist to the right, placing your left hand on your right knee. Turn your head to look to your right, gazing toward or over your right shoulder.
3. Inhale during your twist and try to sit up taller. On your exhale, return to the Mountain pose.
4. Inhale again and gently twist to your left, placing your right hand on your left knee. Notice your breathing as you sit up tall. Exhale and return to the Mountain pose.
5. Repeat this pose five times on each side.

SEATED FORWARD FOLD

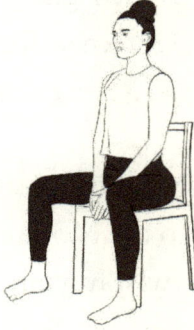

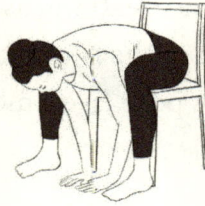

This posture increases the mobility in your back while strengthening the muscles of your lower back. It also provides an incredible stretch for your back, neck, and shoulders.

1. Begin by sitting up tall in your chair with your feet facing forward and firmly on the ground and your palms resting on your thighs.
2. Inhale, and with your back straight, begin to lean forward from your hips as if you're peering into a pond. Only go as far as you can while keeping your back straight.
3. As you exhale, engage the muscles of your core, and using your hands for support, lift back up to a seated position.
4. Repeat this movement at least five times. Your movements may be big or small depending on the flexibility of your spine and the mobility of your hips. Don't worry about it. As you strengthen your muscles, you will increase your flexibility.

BACKBEND

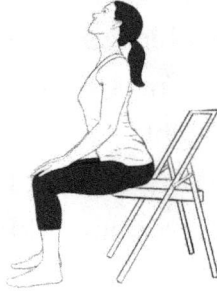

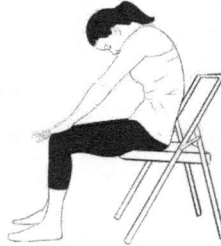

This posture is great for warming up the upper and lower back and is a counterpose to the seated forward fold. It also helps with your posture.

1. Begin in Mountain pose with your palms resting on the tops of your thighs.

2. As you inhale, slowly lift your chin, open your chest and shoulders, and slightly arch your back, looking up at the ceiling.
3. On your exhale, lower your chin to your chest, drop your head, and round your shoulders looking down at the floor.
4. Try to get the movements to flow with your breath. Do this movement at least five times.

SEATED TO CHAIR POSE

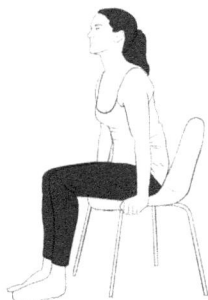

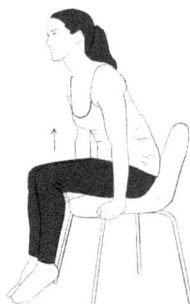

This movement builds strength in the muscles that support you when you're standing and sitting. It also improves your balance.

1. Begin by sitting up in your chair with your knees hip-width apart and your feet on the ground, toes pointing forward. Place your hands on the sides of your chair.
2. Bend forward as if you're going into a Seated Forward Fold, keeping your back and neck straight and in line.
3. Staying in this forward position, slowly lift up from your chair (about six inches) and then lower back down, returning to your seated position.
4. Repeat this pose eight times.

EAGLE ARMS

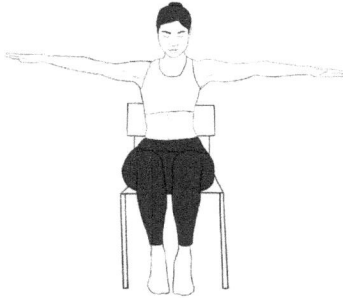

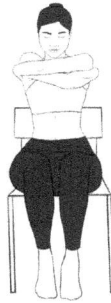

This posture helps to stabilize and flex your shoulder joints while relaxing your upper back and shoulders.

1. To begin, come to the Mountain pose.
2. As you inhale, extend your arms up and out to your sides.

3. As you exhale, bring your arms forward placing your right arm under your left arm and holding your shoulders with opposite hands, as if you're giving yourself a hug. If you have more flexibility in your shoulders, you can keep wrapping your arms until the palms of your hands are touching each other, instead of touching your shoulders.

4. Inhale and lift your arms a little higher. Exhale to release your arms back to your sides.

5. Repeat this movement on the opposite side with your left arm going under your right. Do this pose at least three times.

FULL BODY STRETCH WITH WEIGHTS

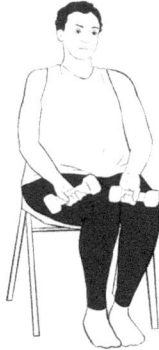

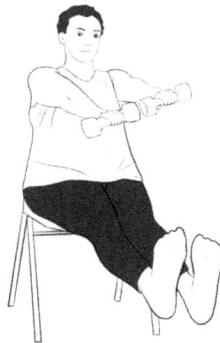

This pose not only strengthens all your muscles, but the addition of weights helps to tone those muscles.

1. Begin in Mountain pose, holding a two-pound weight in each hand, and rest your hands on your thighs.

2. As you breathe in, lift your arms and legs up at the same time. Try to keep your back straight. If you feel like you're slouching, lower your arms and legs a little until you feel like you can stay straight.
3. As you exhale, slowly lower your arms and legs back to your starting position.
4. Repeat this movement eight times. Once you're done, return to the Mountain pose and observe your breath. Notice how your body feels.

6

ADVANCED POSES

These poses require a bit more effort as well as strength and mobility. If you've been practicing for a while you can definitely try these. You can also combine or mix some of the beginner or intermediate poses with these for a slightly more intense practice.

SEATED CAT-COW

This pose helps to relieve tension in your back and shoulders while giving you a great stretch along your spine. It also helps to strengthen the muscles of the back.

1. Begin by sitting up tall in Mountain pose.

2. Inhale and slowly begin to arch your spine, rolling your shoulders back and down.
3. As you breathe out, round your spine, draw your belly in, and bring your chin to your chest.
4. Repeat these movements for five breaths.

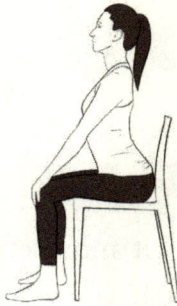

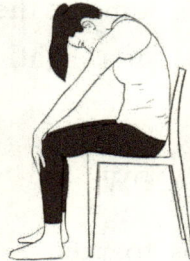

REVERSE ARM HOLD

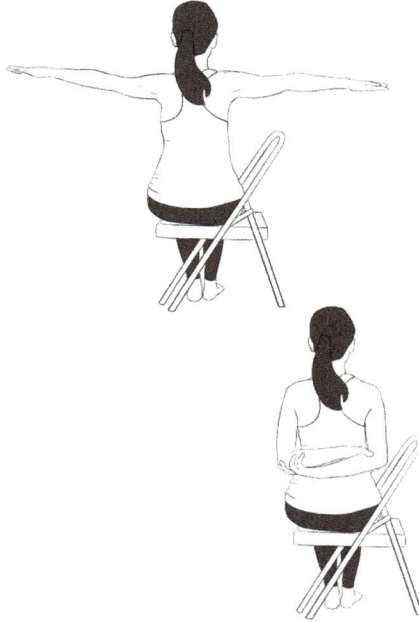

In addition to helping you relax, this pose helps to open up tight shoulders and stretches your chest, increasing mobility and flexibility in your shoulder joints.

1. Begin by sitting up straight with your knees hip-width apart.

2. As you inhale, lift both arms up and out to your sides with the palms facing down.
3. Exhale and gently swing both arms behind you and clasp your elbows with opposite arms. Take three slow breaths here, then release.
4. Repeat the movements, clasping the opposite way.

SEATED LOW LUNGE

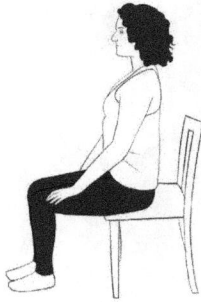

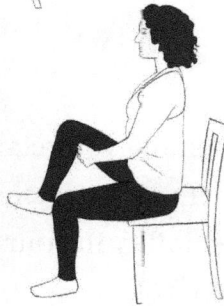

This pose can be restorative and is great for those who have hip pain or tightness in the hips. It strengthens the floor of the pelvis and helps to stabilize your hips.

1. Begin in Mountain pose.
2. Clasp your hands under your right thigh and on an inhale slowly raise your right knee towards your chest. Hold for one breath and release. If you find the pose difficult, sit all the way back in your chair and only lift the knee as far as feels comfortable.
3. Repeat the movement with the left leg. Try to do it at least eight times for each leg.

SEATED WARRIOR I

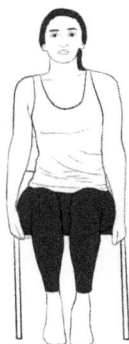

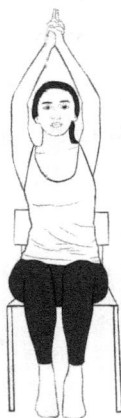

This pose improves circulation in your body and stretches the muscles in your arms.

1. Start in Mountain pose.
2. As you inhale, slowly lift your arms above your head. Interlace your fingers leaving the index

fingers free and pointing up. Take a moment to notice where your shoulders are. Try to relax them down and away from your ears.

3. Take five slow breaths, then release your hands.
4. Repeat this movement five times.

SEATED SIDE ANGLE

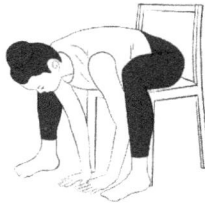

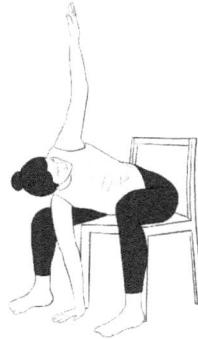

Seated Side Angle engages your core while stretching and strengthening your chest, shoulders, and lungs.

1. Come to a <u>Seated Forward Fold</u> but extend your arms down to the floor.
2. Place your left fingertips on the floor or a block.
3. As you inhale, open your chest and twist to your right lifting your right arm up toward the ceiling. You can look up at your right arm if it feels comfortable. Hold here for three breaths, then release back to your Seated Forward Fold.
4. Repeat with your right fingertips on the floor and your left arm extended.
5. Try to do this movement at least five times on each side.

SEATED PIGEON POSE

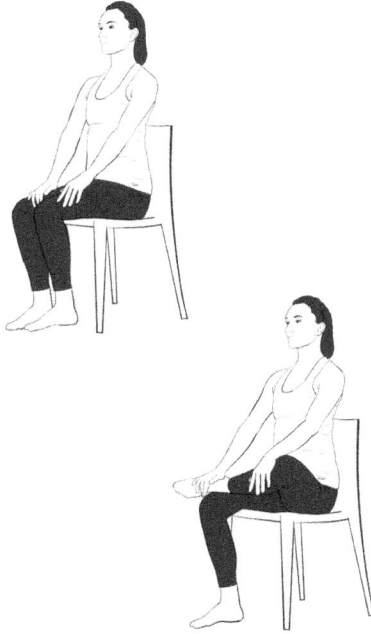

If you suffer from digestive issues this pose can help to alleviate some of the discomfort. It also stretches and strengthens your glutes and groin.

1. Come to sitting straight with your feet firmly planted on the floor, knees hip-distance apart and toes pointing forward.

2. Bring your right ankle up and place it on your left knee. Try not to let your left leg collapse inward.
3. Hold this pose for five breaths, then repeat with the other leg.
4. Do this at least three times for each leg.

FIVE-POINT STAR

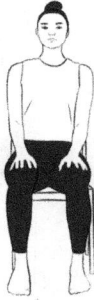

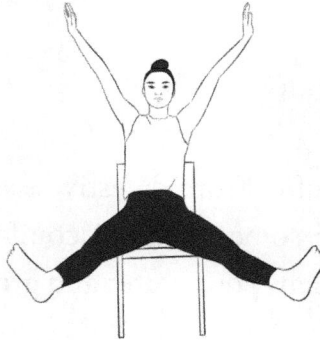

This pose is fantastic for your posture. It aligns, strengthens, and lengthens your spine. Not to mention, it's a great total body stretch.

1. Begin in Mountain pose.
2. On an inhale, extend your arms and legs out at the same time to create a star shape. If extending your arms and legs at the same time is difficult, do the arms first and then the legs. Remember, only go as far as feels right to you.
3. Exhale and release back to Mountain pose.
4. Complete this pose three times.

CHAIR CORPSE POSE

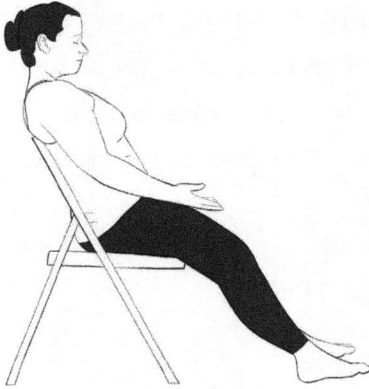

This is just about the best way to end your practice, refocus on yourself and notice your breath.

1. From your seated position, lean back in your chair, extend your legs out in front of you, and let your arms rest loose at your sides.
2. Close your eyes and simply observe your breath and the sensations. You can practice your meditation at this point if you would like.

CONCLUSION

Yoga is not only about caring for the physical body. It seeks to create harmony and balance between the mind, body, and spirit. You can practice yoga anywhere, at any time simply by taking a few moments to connect with your breath and notice how you're feeling.

Yoga can help to relax or calm you in stressful situations and it can make you stronger and more independent in your daily activities. Yoga is not just to be practiced on your chair but in your life.

The tools and poses that have been shared in this book are just stepping stones for you to lead a healthier, happier, calmer, and more independent life. As you begin or continue your yoga journey, try to remain consistent and persistent. Patience and steadiness are part of your yoga practice, so include them in your daily life. Above all else, enjoy it.

REFERENCES

Carraco, M. (2007, August 28). *A beginner's guide to meditation*. Yoga Journal. https://www.yogajournal.com/meditation/how-to-meditate/let-s-meditate/

Cherry, K. (2020, September 1). *What is meditation?* Verywell Mind. https://www.verywellmind.com/what-is-meditation-2795927

Cohut, M. (2017, August 27). *How yoga, meditation benefit the mind and body*. Www.medicalnewstoday.com. https://www.medicalnewstoday.com/articles/319116

Cronkleton, E. (2021, April 14). *Yoga for osteoporosis: 5 beneficial poses & how to do them*. Healthline. https://www.healthline.com/health/osteoporosis/yoga-for-osteoporosis#1

Ekhart, E. (2014, June 25). *The importance of breath in yoga*. Ekhart Yoga. https://www.ekhartyoga.com/articles/practice/the-importance-of-breath-in-yoga

Hastings, C. (2017, August 2). *Science shows yoga may protect your brain in old age*. World Economic Forum. https://www.weforum.org/agenda/2017/08/science-shows-yoga-may-protect-your-brain-in-old-age

REFERENCES

Hullet, A. (2020, August 27). *Take a seat: 11 chair yoga poses to try.* Greatist. https://greatist.com/move/chair-yoga?c=643257173729#11-chair-yoga-poses-to-try

Lehmkuhl, L. (2020). *Chair yoga for seniors: Stretches and poses that you can do sitting down at home.* Skyhorse Publishing.

McGee, K. (2017, March 30). *Chair yoga meditation: Stillness as a complement to movement. Kristin McGee.* https://kristinmcgee.com/chair-yoga-meditation

Nichols, H. (2021, April 14). *Yoga: Methods, types, philosophy, and risks.* Www.medicalnewstoday.com. https://www.medicalnewstoday.com/articles/286745

Stelter, G. (2015, December 7). *Chair yoga for seniors: Seated poses.* Healthline. https://www.healthline.com/health/fitness-exercise/chair-yoga-for-seniors

Yoga Anytime. (2019, August 23). *Yoga breathing 101: Beginner tips and practices.* Yoga Anytime. https://www.yogaanytime.com/blog/meditation/yoga-breathing-101-beginner-tips-and-practices

BALANCE EXERCISES FOR SENIORS

EASY EXERCISES TO PERFORM AT HOME THAT HELP
PREVENT FALLS AND INJURIES

FIT FOREVER

FIT FOREVER

INTRODUCTION

I am sure you would like to be able to do the things you once did when you were younger. Getting older can be scary when our balance isn't what it used to be, and falls can have disastrous effects.

But in a world that promotes strenuous exercise and marathon-running bodies, it can be daunting to want to try to get fit, especially knowing that you can't do those kinds of exercises.

You have taken a great first step in wanting to see what else is available to you. This book is going to introduce you to different types of exercises and stretching techniques. These exercises are geared towards not just your fitness level but also your mobility level, so everyone is catered for. What's more, they are explained in detail so that they are easy to follow starting from beginner to advanced, and they also explain the various benefits you will get.

You will see that your life will change for the better, and you will find yourself being able to enjoy life as you should.

To get the most out of this book, stay consistent with the exercises, and work within your comfort zone. Listen to your body, and move at your own pace.

It is important to note that this is a self-published book. Only you and your healthcare team know your body's limits. Therefore, before you start any exercise, it is advisable to consult your doctor first.

1

THE BENEFITS OF EXERCISE

When you start exercising it can be difficult to grasp the full range of benefits your body and mind will experience because these can only be felt and seen over time.

It is important to remain focused on how much freedom you are going to gain once you are more mobile. Think about how nice it will be not to be trapped at home, afraid of falling, or encumbered with aches and pains.

Exercise at any age is beneficial—both mentally and physically—but as we age, it becomes even more important to prevent our mobility from deteriorating to a point that we lose our independence. We need to be fit to keep on living independently without the help of others for as long as possible.

MENTAL BENEFITS

Physical activity has been known to produce endorphins that help you feel good and combat stress. Exercise puts you in a happier state of mind to help you deal with life's everyday issues. You start to become more confident and sure of yourself which increases your quality of life.

Cognitive Improvement

Exercise helps to improve deteriorating motor skills and this, in turn, is great for dementia prevention in the long term. Physical activity improves your ability to multitask and increases your creativity over time.

Better Sleep

Your quality of sleep starts to deteriorate in old age which can lead to a string of mental health problems. Exercise helps you to relax, creates physical fatigue, and thus, helps you sleep better at night. It also helps prevent insomnia and promotes deeper better-quality sleep over time. This, in turn, allows you to wake up refreshed and full of energy to embark on your day-to-day activities.

Hobby Maintenance

A lot of us have numerous hobbies, and this amount grows as we get older, retire, and have the time to spend on them. Hobbies keep our wits sharp and give meaning to the every-day. When our muscles and joints become stiff and prevent us from doing those hobbies, it can lead to psychological damage and depression. Exercise helps keep our moving parts workable so that we can continue to enjoy our hobbies without pain and discomfort.

Social Activity

Isolation increases the risk of depression from loneliness, so it's important to remain social as we get older. Exercise is a fun activity that can be done as a group and expands an older person's social circle. Various exercise classes are available that are geared towards seniors, and they can not *just* provide great ways of staying fit but also offer added social interactions.

PHYSICAL BENEFITS

Increased Flexibility

As we get older, our joints become stiff, and that impacts our flexibility. Osteoarthritic pain is also a common issue that causes muscles and joints to get so stiff that mobility becomes painful. Exercises will help ease this pain and maintain flexibility because they work on strengthening the surrounding muscles. Inflammation is also decreased, as lubrication increases in our joints when exercising regularly.

Lowers the Risk of Falling

Falling can be fatal in old age, as we often hurt ourselves so badly that the necessary healing can be extensive or even out of reach. Exercises targeting balance and muscle strength help to prevent falling by increasing mobility and flexibility in our muscles and joints.

Weight Loss and Maintenance

Most people start to put on more weight as they get older because their metabolism slows down. This can increase the chance of several chronic diseases, like heart disease and diabetes. Regular physical activity will help to increase metabolism in older adults so that a healthy weight can be maintained.

Immunity Boost

Our immunity also starts to decline as we age, but regular exercise can help boost immunity and speed up recovery from illnesses. This is because physical activity helps white blood cells to circulate faster to detect illnesses and work on fighting these off in the body.

Likewise, stress hormones can bring about illness but exercise helps to lower the release of these hormones.

Bone Density Increase

Our bones start to weaken with age, and some older adults may develop osteoporosis because of this. This makes bones so weak that fractures could easily occur. Physical activity helps with improving bone density and maintaining strength for years to come. Your bones consist of living tissue that responds to the pressure put on it. That's why consistent exercise helps your bones become denser over time.

Chronic Disease Prevention

Diseases like colon cancer, diabetes, obesity, osteoporosis, hypertension, and heart disease are just some of the conditions that can start occurring in old age. Physical activity helps build up the immune system which, in turn, helps to prevent or manage these diseases better as we get older.

For people that already have these chronic diseases, exercise helps with minimizing the symptoms. This makes managing the disease much easier and increases one's quality of life

2

CONSISTENCY

We often want quick solutions to our problems and become quite impatient to see results. Exercise can exacerbate these feelings of impatience because the benefits are felt over time and with consistency. It's not a quick fix to increase one's mobility.

If physical activity is done too often and for long periods in an attempt to get quick results, it will lead to injury. This is because you end up doing too much for a few days, and then, stopping for weeks. Your body and muscles start to experience fatigue or are working so hard that they get injured.

Starting off slow and at your own pace is a step in the right direction. In time, you will be able to exercise for longer and do more complicated exercises. The aim is to progressively build up strength and flexibility.

By remaining consistent you will create an exercise habit, and it will start to become easier to exercise. You will notice that you start to want to do physical activity rather than thinking it to be a chore.

By exercising at a consistent pace, you will also notice that the pain and soreness experienced from exercise will start to decrease as you become stronger.

WHY IS IT SO HARD TO BE CONSISTENT?

When we try something new, we do so with a burst of energy and high expectations of the results. We start off excited and enthusiastic but often expect too much too soon.

Once we start to realize that we are not reaching the targets we set, or have missed a few goals, we feel demotivated and eventually stop completely.

Consistency is all about behavioral changes and good habit forming. That is why it takes time and effort.

To be consistent, you need to embrace that it is a lifestyle change—the lifestyle of wanting to be healthy and living a healthy life. For something to become a habit over time, it needs to stop being a conscious thought, instead becoming something that you carry out naturally or automatically, like brushing your teeth or tying your shoelaces. You don't think about doing these tasks, you do them subconsciously, but you had to have learned them first. A habit was created over time.

Exercise is often seen as something one needs to do, a task that takes effort and is not enjoyable. This makes us consciously think about it often and, hence, come up with reasons to miss exercise days. We might even create a negative experience around exercise to the point that we hate doing it and would rather stop altogether.

HOW CAN WE CREATE A GOOD HABIT?

Habit forming takes time and commitment, but it helps to follow a plan so you can stay on track.

Keep Track

Tracking the progress you are making is very helpful in getting a habit to stick. You can choose to use one of the many free apps available on your phone or simply use a notebook and a pen. Write down the habit and each day's progress. If you miss a day, note that with the reason. This will help you to overcome things that are preventing you from achieving your daily goal. It will also help you to be accountable for days missed.

Check Your Motivation

That initial burst of enthusiasm doesn't count as motivation. Staying motivated about exercise is about what you hope to achieve, and only once you truly know this will you be fully prepared to be consistent to get there.

Ask yourself why you need to exercise: What ails you that exercise will solve? How will your life change for the better because of physical activity? Take the time to explore your reasoning, and then, use this as a daily reminder to keep yourself motivated.

The Cycle of Habits

Habits are formed via a cycle:

1. Trigger

This is what commences the habit like an alarm going off to remind you to start exercising. The trigger should be automatic but also something noticeable enough to prompt you. The aim is for your reaction to the trigger to be subconscious, not something that takes effort.

2. Routine

This is the physical activity you need to do because the trigger has reminded you. So, in this case, you would get dressed and prepare for doing some physical activity. It's important to complete this set of tasks in the same way each time.

3. Reward

This is the sense of achievement that helps to keep you motivated towards continuing the habit. For example, the act of exercising has given you more energy. Without a reward, you won't feel the act of exercising is worth it.

For this cycle to operate at an optimum level, it will take some time and requires that you stay consistent and consciously make the effort.

Focus On Adding Not Subtracting

The biggest mistake most people make when trying to create a new habit is to try to stop the bad habits at the same time. This takes far too much effort because you will be thinking of too many things at once. It's a technique that will doom you to failure.

Just focus on the good habit, and keep it simple. In time, as you naturally enjoy the good habit, and it becomes routine, you will notice the bad habits stop without you having to overthink it or make any extra effort.

One Step at a Time

To form a habit, we need to be focused on taking one step at a time. If we have too many things going on, it becomes too much to mentally juggle and causes the habit to not take hold. With exercise, start with basic exercises appropriate to your fitness level and mobility. Focus on keeping to an exercise schedule each week, and in time, you will see how easy it is to keep. Then, you can shift your focus to increasing your fitness levels.

3

THE REASONS SENIORS FALL

Aging is a natural process that happens to all of us. It is both psychosocial and biological. Psychosocial, because our societal roles start to change. We may be retired and, therefore, have different goals and priorities in life as we get older. From a biological perspective, every part of our body starts to change, even the smallest of cells. This means we lose strength, balance, and flexibility over time.

All these changes mean that as we get older, falling can become a lot more common. The risk is greater than just getting bruised, as senior falls can lead to head injuries, hip fractures, or even broken bones. These types of injuries take away one's ability to live alone or be able to do their day-to-day tasks with ease.

Even when the falls don't cause serious injury, they cause older adults to become fearful, and so, they start cutting down on their normal activities. This has the knock-on effect of making them weaker over time and increasing their chances of injury from falling.

There are various reasons that falling starts to become a risk as we get older:

- Lightheadedness is caused by low blood pressure.
- Our vision starts to deteriorate causing us to miss objects that used to be clear.
- Stumbling is caused by not being able to lift our feet off the ground as we used to.
- Incorrect footwear is often being used.
- Vitamin D deficiencies are common.
- Long-term use of certain medications can lead to a loss of balance or dizziness.
- Leg muscles and hip joints start to lose strength.
- Slow reaction times, especially to objects in our way, cause us to trip and fall easily.
- Medical conditions like postural hypotension, arthritis, vestibular disorders, strokes, multiple sclerosis, diabetes, Parkinson's disease, and dementia impact balance.
- Some people develop spinal degeneration or develop a poor posture that affects their posture and ability to remain stable.

Falls can be prevented, and that's where exercise plays a huge part. It helps to keep older adults steady on their feet to avoid falls or recover faster.

HOW EXERCISE HELPS WITH FALLING

Our balance deteriorates over time, but this is mostly due to inactivity. Therefore, keeping and maintaining one's balance has a lot to do with movement and exercise.

Exercise that consists of balance training, strength training, and endurance training will help you build strength in your muscles, and you will start to become more mobile and able to maintain balance. This, in turn, improves your overall balance which decreases your chances of falling and could even lead to quicker recovery should you fall.

As your balance starts to improve, so does your confidence and your ability to react to objects and situations to prevent falls from occurring. This ability is called balance recovery reaction and is something we take for granted when we are younger because it's an automatic movement. When we get older, we need to retrain ourselves to react this way like grabbing hold of a surface close by or using our feet to step out and regain balance.

The confidence gained from balance improvement also aids in fall prevention and helps to improve one's posture, consequently helping to maintain balance.

Balance-Specific Exercises

Your base of support is the place under your feet that makes contact with the floor. Venturing outside of this space without wobbling and falling is an indicator of good balance.

Balance exercises are aimed at improving that reach for older adults and being reactive. As a result, some exercises are geared towards losing balance and getting it back again, but only in a safe way that is managed.

4

THE SCIENCE BEHIND BALANCE

I n science, we are considered to be balanced when our body is in a state of equilibrium. Very simply, this means when all forces pushing down on us are equal to our ability to push back. This ability to push back is based on our potential to distribute our mass evenly.

We often take our balance for granted when we are young, because we have natural balance, and often, only wonder consider it if we happen to trip or fall.

Balance becomes a bigger issue as we get older because we start to lose what we took for granted for so long. Surgeries, reliance on long-term medication, and muscle loss due to less activity all contribute to our loss of balance. Consequently, that leads to an increased risk of falling and the dangers that could bring to an aging body.

BALANCE EXPLAINED

We can remain steady and upright because balance allows for our weight to be distributed evenly. For this to work effectively three different body systems need to work together:

- Vestibular system: Found in the inner ear, this allows us to sense where our body and the head are while we are moving.
- Vision Systems: These allow us to keep our sight stable while we move.
- Proprioception: The ability to know where our body is in relation to gravity keeps us aware of our surroundings.

Balance is all to do with how different body systems and functions are communicating with the brain so that certain muscles can move efficiently. It's a complex array of systems that need to work and talk to each other clearly so that we can step over obstacles, sit down, walk up stairs, avoid an object in our path, or even stand up.

There is a reason that as children we are told to stop, look, *and* listen before crossing the road; our bodies require various stimuli to keep us aware of potential dangers and the safety of movement. Our senses send signals throughout this process so that, with each movement, we maintain our balance.

Not all circumstances call for every system to be working at the same time though, often just one or two is required. Regardless, all aspects of balance need to be strengthened as we get older to ensure we can be balanced in every possible situation.

The fluid-filled canals in our inner ears communicate our position to our brains so they can identify whether we are standing, sitting, or lying down. These also measure where our bodies are in relation to the earth's gravity.

Our hips, ankles, and knees also send sensory information to the brain.

If any one of these systems stops working, our base of support is compromised and our balance is thrown off, allowing falls to occur.

5

TYPES OF EXERCISES

I n this chapter, I am going to include the different types of exercises that will be used in this book and the benefits of each one.

VESTIBULAR EXERCISES

Also called *Balance Exercises*, these are aimed at helping to bring back equilibrium to your body by building up the muscles. Over time, these exercises help you rebuild strength.

It is important to note that dizziness will be felt to varying degrees, but it shouldn't be a concern.

How Do They Work?

Vestibular exercises are designed to help the brain shift its outlook on abnormalities or injuries to help bring about balance. They train the brain to not restrain you as you exercise and see it as positive stimulation rather than a cause for concern.

Eye movement is taught independent of head movement creating muscle sense awareness over time. This allows the body to learn how to regain balance in various situations.

You will be exposed to a lot of movements that cause dizziness at first, but as time goes on, you will regain your confidence doing any movement—even spontaneous ones—and not be afraid of being mobile, even in the dark.

It is recommended that you keep up these exercises, and try not to relapse. Start very slowly, and in time, increase the speed of each movement, also trying for longer repetitions, if possible.

SEATED EXERCISES

These types of exercises are great for beginners but can also get more complex while still offering support.

By sitting on a chair, lower and upper body exercises help to concentrate on the muscles in your legs and arms. The chair also supports your back and helps you to get into a good posture that can then be maintained easier.

Chair exercises incorporate stretching, using the full range of motion available to you, starting from what you are comfortable with to a full-body workout. The chair provides added balance and stability so you can be confident of not falling.

Blood circulation is improved and an increased heart rate occurs to guarantee a proper workout that doesn't require you to do anything strenuous. You will also feel an energy increase.

Muscle strength and flexibility are improved, and the joints start to become more lubricated which also helps to reduce any stress and anxiety you have been experiencing.

STANDING EXERCISES

These exercises are aimed at seniors who are not as frail and have a better balance or use a walking stick sufficiently to get around.

Standing exercises are focused on building up core strength to create and maintain stability. Some standing exercises also help you to test your balance levels so you can gauge if you need to increase your fitness level.

Specific standing exercises can improve balance with controlled movements specific to different aspects of balance.

MOVING/WALKING EXERCISES

Even though you are not running, these types of exercises still count as cardio. You will find that your energy increases and your circulatory system improves.

By moving—no matter how slow—you are testing and building up your ability to balance yourself. These also help improve confidence in walking and climbing stairs.

CORE EXERCISES

Our core muscles are found right in the center of our bodies and reach down to our hips, spine, buttocks, and pelvis. Without them we can't stand, sit, stay balanced, bend, or even lift anything up.

Strengthening these muscles is very important for balance in seniors to improve posture and increase mobility. A lot of core exercises can be done either sitting or standing, depending on your fitness level and mobility.

The core exercises found in this book not only help to strengthen your core but also assist with pain management, especially when it comes to lower back pain. In time, with consistency, the pain will start to reduce.

EQUIPMENT NEEDED

For most of the exercises—especially the beginner exercises —a sturdy chair will be needed. Make sure that the chair has a back for support and is armless with no wheels. Dining room or kitchen chairs work fine for this, but you don't want to be using an unstable plastic chair.

Wear comfortable shoes that are not slippery or able to come off when exercising. No sandals or high heels should be used to exercise. Use well-cushioned shoes that are comfortable but also offer added support.

Don't wear tight clothing that will impair movement; wear loose comfortable clothing. Keep a bottle of water close by to take regular sips during exercise breaks.

CONSIDER THE FOLLOWING

Don't exercise if you are not well. Even if you have a slight cold, it is best to get over the illness completely before undertaking any physical activity.

You will naturally feel muscle and joint pain after exercising, but the intensity of this pain is worth noting. If it is very uncomfortable, then lower your exercise intensity, and speak to your doctor should the pain persist.

6

BEGINNER EXERCISES

A ll of these exercises require the use of a sturdy chair so that you have support as you do each move.

Always start with the warm-up exercise. Don't skip this as it will help ease you into the exercises that follow and put you in the right headspace.

If you start to feel dizzy, stop and rest. When you start again, slow down your movements and be sure to breathe deeply. If you are struggling to complete any of the exercises, move on to the next one.

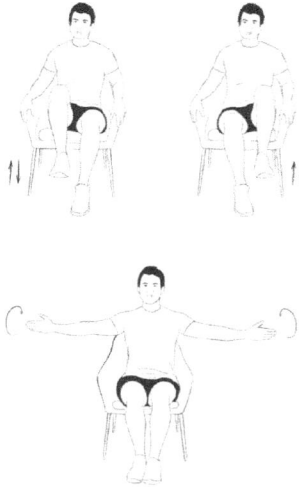

WARM UP

1. Sit back on your chair, legs slightly apart and with your arms down each side of the chair.
2. Pick your right leg up, and then set it down.
3. Pick your left leg up, and set it down.
4. March like this—while sitting—for 60 seconds, breathing deeply in and out.
5. Rest both your feet on the floor.
6. Move your arms to the sides.
7. Make circles with your arms, in a clockwise direction, for 60 seconds.
8. Slowly, drop your arms back down to each side of the chair.

9. Repeat the marching and arm circles two more times.

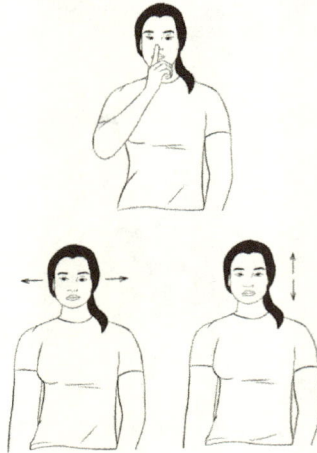

EYE EXERCISES

1. Sit back straight and comfortably on your chair.
2. Keep your feet firmly on the ground with your head still and facing forward.
3. Place your right index finger on the tip of your nose, and look at it for 10 seconds.
4. Look directly forward, and then, move your eyes from side to side for 10 seconds.
5. Move your eyes up and down for 10 seconds.
6. Return to the starting position, and repeat 19 more times.

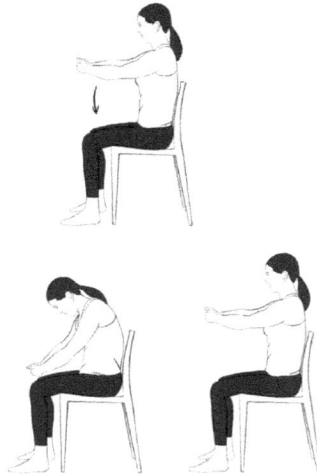

HALFWAY BACK-ROLLS

1. Sit straight with your back firmly on the backrest of your chair.
2. Keep your feet on the ground with your knees bent.
3. Slowly lift your arms in front of you, without slouching or leaning back.
4. Turn your hands so that your fingers interlock and you create a circle with your arms.
5. Slowly bring in your tummy as you round your back.
6. Go as far as you can, and hold for 10 seconds.
7. Roll yourself back to the starting position.
8. Repeat four more times.

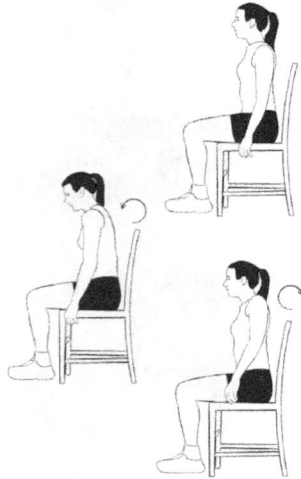

SHOULDER EXERCISES

1. Sit back straight and comfortably on your chair.
2. Face forward.
3. Rotate your shoulder to the left and then to the right.
4. Repeat this 19 times.
5. Return to the starting sitting position, facing forward.
6. Keep your arms to your side, and with each breath, shrug your shoulders at least 20 times.

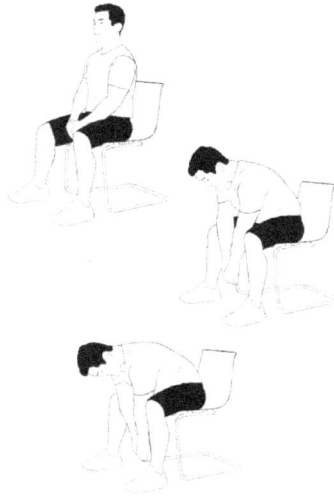

FORWARD BENDS

1. Sit back straight and comfortably on your chair.
2. Bend your body forward as though to touch the ground. Reach as far as you can comfortably go.
3. Sit back up, and concentrate on moving your eyes down to the floor and back up for 20 seconds.
4. Repeat 19 more times.
5. Once again, bend your body forward as though to touch the ground. Reach as far as you can comfortably go.
6. Sit back up, and focus on an object in front of you for 10 seconds.
7. Repeat this 19 more times.

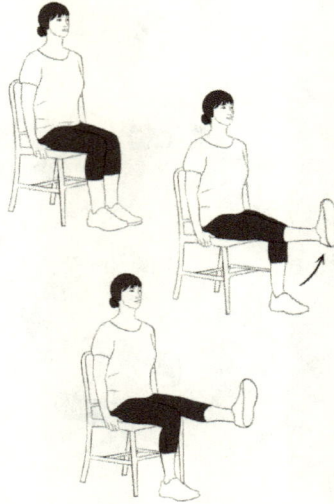

LEG LIFTS

1. Sit with a straight and upright posture to avoid any back-leaning or slouching.
2. Bend your right knee while keeping your right foot on the ground.
3. Extend your left leg, and try to raise it as high as you can while maintaining your straight posture.
4. Hold for five seconds, and then, bring your left leg down so that the left foot is on the ground.
5. Bend your left knee while keeping your left foot on the ground.
6. Extend your right leg, and try to raise it as high as you can while maintaining your straight posture. 7. Hold for five seconds, and then, bring your right leg

down so that the right foot is on the ground. 8. Repeat twice more on both sides.

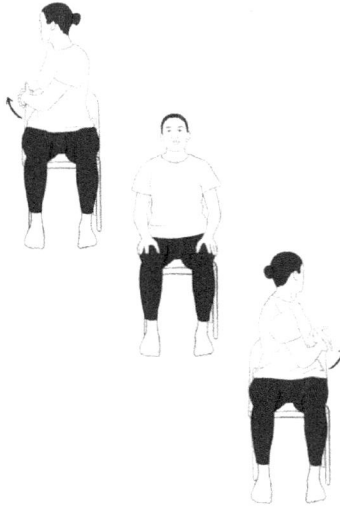

ROTATIONS

1. Sit back straight and comfortably on your chair.
2. Face forward, and close your eyes.
3. Rotate your entire upper body to the right, keeping your eyes closed, and hold for 10 seconds.
4. Return to the forward position, and repeat 19 more times.
5. Open your eyes.
6. Rotate your upper body to the left, keeping your eyes open, and hold for 10 seconds.

7. Return to the starting position, and repeat 19 more times.

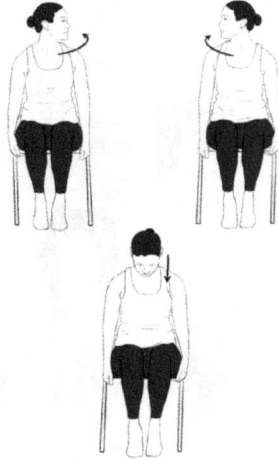

HEAD ROTATION WHILE SITTING

1. Sit straight with your back firmly on the backrest of your chair.
2. Keep your spine as straight as you can manage. Your arms must be to the sides of the chair and your feet slightly apart.
3. Stare straight ahead.
4. Slowly move your head to the right, then the left, and lastly, tilt your head downward.
5. Repeat 9 more times.

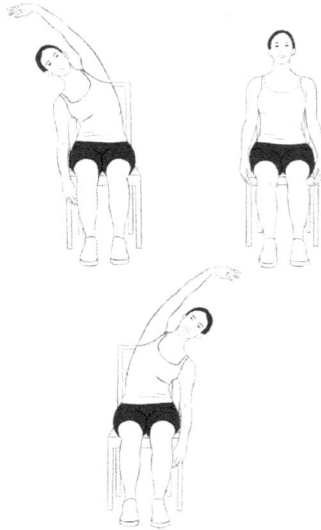

SIDE BENDS WHILE SEATED

1. Sit in the upright position in your chair, sitting all the way back.
2. Keep your legs together and your feet flat on the ground. Your arms must be to the sides of the chair.
3. Bend your left arm up so that your left hand is resting on the side of your head, over your ear.
4. Let your right arm hang to the side, but keep your posture straight.
5. Take a deep breath in, and hold it for five seconds.
6. As you exhale, slowly bend your right arm and waist down so that you are leaning towards the floor on your right side.

7. Keep your elbow back to feel that stretch if you are able to, holding for five seconds.
8. Return to the forward position.
9. Bend your right arm so that your right hand is resting on the side of your head, over your ear.
10. Let your left arm hang to the side, but keep your posture straight.
11. Take a deep breath in, and hold it for five seconds.
12. As you exhale, slowly bend your left arm and waist down so that you are leaning towards the floor on your left side.
13. Keep your elbow back to feel that stretch if you are able to, holding for five seconds.
14. Return to the forward position.
15. Do this 3 times on each side.

7

INTERMEDIATE EXERCISES

Some of these exercises require that you stand near or facing a wall for support. Other exercises require a sturdy chair.

Start with the warm-up exercise. Don't skip it as it will help to ease you into the exercises in this chapter and put you in the right headspace.

Should you start to feel dizzy, stop and rest. When you start again, slow down your movements and be sure to breathe deeply. If you are struggling to complete any of the exercises, move on to the next one.

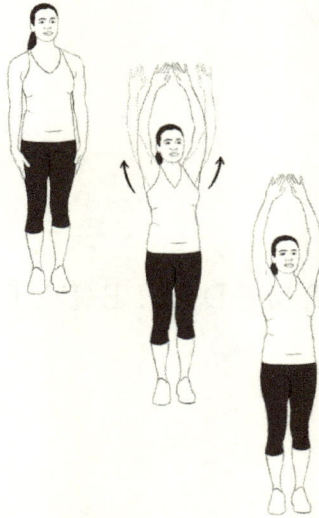

WARM UP

1. Stand up straight facing a wall for support or next to a study chair.
2. Take a deep breath in.
3. Breathe out as you lift your arms slowly above your head.
4. Hold that stretch for 20 seconds.
5. Bring your arms slowly down.
6. Repeat four more times.

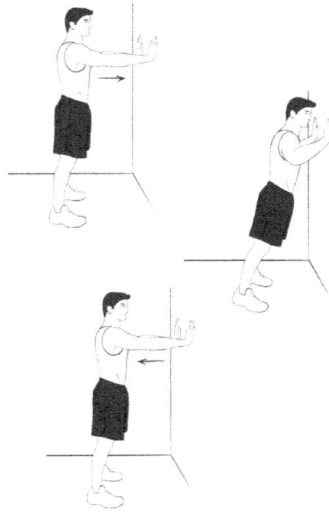

PUSH-UPS USING A WALL

1. Stand up straight, facing a wall at arm's length.
2. Place your arms, at shoulder height, against the wall. Your palms must be flat against the wall.
3. Your feet must be slightly apart and also flat on the ground.
4. Lean toward the wall, as you would do a push-up.
5. Move back, and repeat 19 more times.

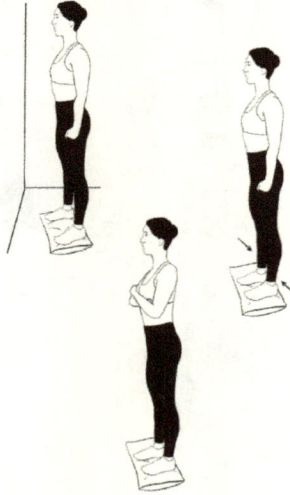

CUSHION STANDING

1. Stand on a cushion while facing a wall for support.
2. Try not to grab the wall if you can avoid it, and hold your body straight for 30 seconds.
3. Keep your eyes open while you do this. If you start to feel dizzy, then keep your eyes closed.
4. Step off the cushion.

As you progress to doing this without wobbling and needing the wall for support, increase intensity in two ways:

- Keep your feet closer together on the cushion.
- Cross your arms over your chest.

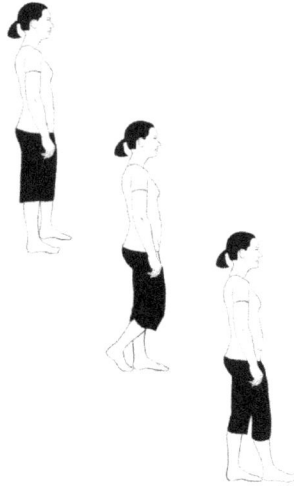

HEEL TO TOE

1. Stand up, feet slightly apart, facing a wall.
2. Place one foot in front of the other. The front foot's heel must be touching the toe of the back foot.
3. Keep your eyes open, and focus on the wall for 30 seconds.
4. If you feel dizzy or off balance, you can touch the wall to get back into position.
5. After 30 seconds, close your eyes for an additional 30 seconds.
6. Repeat 19 more times.

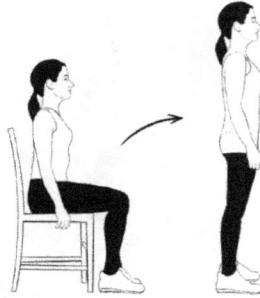

ALTERNATE BETWEEN SITTING AND STANDING

1. Start in a sitting position on a chair that is supporting your back and with your feet firmly on the ground.
2. Keep your eyes open, staring straight ahead for 10 seconds.
3. Slowly get up and stand in front of your chair with your eyes closed for 10 seconds.
4. Repeat this 19 more times.

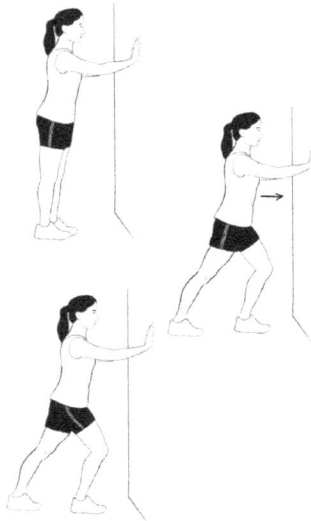

STRETCHING THE CALVES

1. Stand up straight facing a wall for support, allowing yourself space of just over an arm's length.
2. Raise your arms straight until they are at your eye level.
3. Slowly move your right leg behind your left leg. Your right leg heel must be firm on the ground while you do this.
4. Start to bend your left knee but don't go all the way down.
5. Hold for 30 seconds.
6. Return to the starting position.
7. Raise your arms straight so that they are at your eye level.

8. Slowly move your left leg behind your right leg. Your left leg heel must be firm on the ground while you do this.
9. Start to bend your right knee but don't go all the way down.
10. Hold for 30 seconds.
11. Repeat four more times on each side.

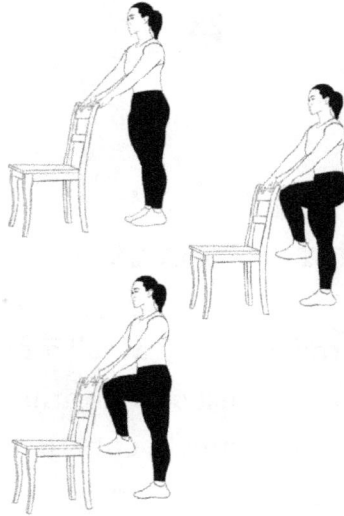

THE ONE LIMB POSE

1. Stand next to your chair, and hold onto the top for support.
2. Lift your left leg up slightly off the ground, and balance on your right foot.
3. Hold for at least 30 seconds.

4. Gently lower your left foot, and repeat with the right foot.
5. Do this for 10 repetitions.

You can try this pose for longer on each side as you get more comfortable and balanced. Aim for not needing the chair and holding this position for a full minute on each leg.

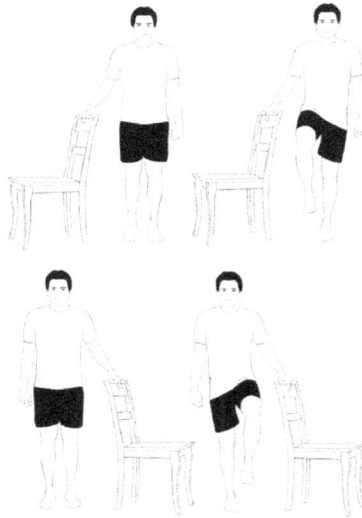

LEG STANDS

1. Stand up straight next to a sturdy chair. The chair must be on your right side.
2. Hold onto the top of the chair with your right hand.
3. Stand on your left leg, with your right leg lifted.
4. Hold this for up to one minute.

5. Lower your right leg.
6. Turn around.
7. Hold onto the top of the chair with your left hand.
8. Stand on your right leg, with your left leg lifted.
9. Hold for up to one minute.
10. Lower your left leg.
11. Repeat 10 more times on each side.

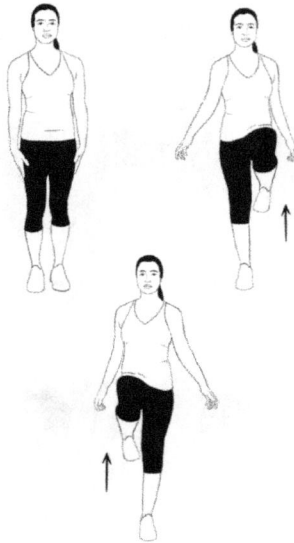

STAND LIKE A FLAMINGO

1. Stand up straight next to a wall or chair.
2. Gently transfer your weight to your left foot.
3. Slowly lift your right foot, and extend that leg forward the way flamingos stand.

4. Stay in this position as long as you can, initially aiming for 15 seconds.
5. Slowly, move your right foot down and straighten up.
6. Shake out your legs.
7. Gently transfer your weight to your right foot.
8. Slowly lift your left foot, and extend that leg forward the way flamingos stand.
9. Stay in this position as long as you can but aim for 15 seconds.
10. Slowly, move your left foot down and straighten up.
11. Shake out your legs.
12. Do this 3 more times on each leg.

8

ADVANCED EXERCISES

I n this chapter, one exercise requires the use of your bed, while another calls for a stool, step, or similar. The rest of these exercises require that you move or walk, often without the use of walls or chairs for support. However, you can still make use of these should you feel you want the support to be there just in case.

These advanced exercises can *only* be done if you have mastered the beginner and intermediate exercises first.

Remember to always start with the warm-up exercise. Skipping it will not help you to ease into the exercises or put you in the right headspace.

If you start to feel dizzy, stop and rest. Then, start again slowly and breathe deeply. If you are struggling to complete any of the exercises, move on to the next one.

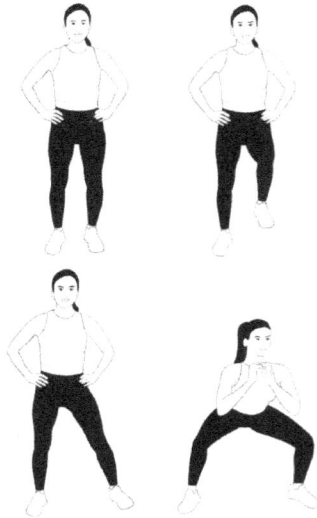

WARM UP

1. Stand up straight with your feet shoulder-width apart.
2. Place your hands on your hips.
3. Transfer your weight to your right leg, and lift your left leg so that your thigh is parallel to the ground.
4. As you bring that left leg down, move it towards the left like you are stepping over something.
5. Once you lower your left leg fully, slowly go into a squat. If a full squat is too much, then aim for a half squat. Hold for 10 seconds.
6. Slowly bring yourself up to the starting position.
7. Transfer your weight to your left leg and lift your right leg so that your thigh is parallel to the ground.

8. As you bring that right leg down, move it towards the right like you are stepping over something.
9. Once you lower your right leg down, slowly go into a squat. If a full squat is too much, then aim for a half squat. Hold for 10 seconds.
10. Slowly bring yourself up to the starting position.
11. Repeat three more times on each side.

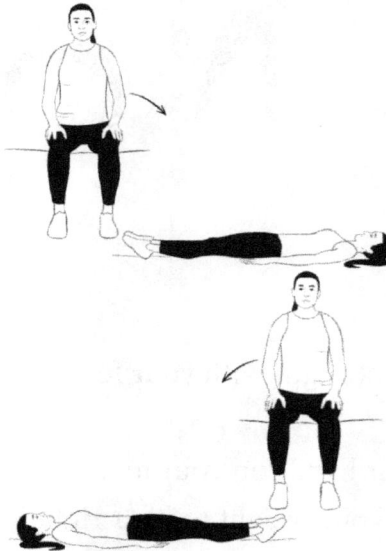

LYING DOWN

1. Sit on the side of your bed in an upright position.
2. Quickly swing your feet onto the bed on the right side and lie down.
3. Breathe deeply for 30 seconds.
4. Slowly, sit back up.

5. Repeat on the other side.
6. Do this twice more on each side.

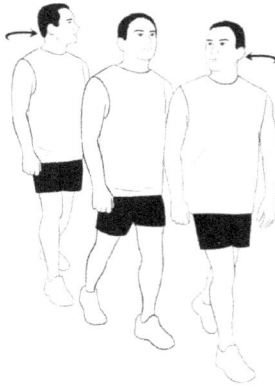

HEAD-TURNING WITH STRAIGHT-LINE WALKING

1. Stand up straight next to a long wall, preferably a hallway.
2. Walk slowly in a straight line while turning your head and eyes to the right and then the left with each breath.
3. Do this for five minutes then stop to rest.
4. Repeat two more times.
5. Start slowly walking again, this time moving your eyes down to the floor and then up to the ceiling as you walk.

6. Repeat two more times.

If the wall is not long enough, stop at the end and turn around. If need to, use the wall for support.

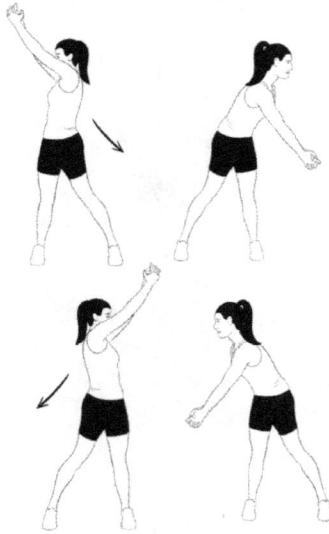

CHOPPING WOOD

1. Stand up straight, at arm's length from a sturdy chair or wall in case you need support.
2. Make sure your feet are flat on the ground and hip-width apart.
3. Move your arms straight in front of you at eye level.
4. Clasp your hands together.
5. Swing your clasped hands down towards your left hip like you are chopping wood.

6. Move your clasped hands up to your right ear.
7. Move back into the initial hands-clasped position.
8. Swing your clasped hands down towards your right hip like you are chopping wood.
9. Move your clasped hands up to your left ear.
10. Move back into the starting position.
11. Repeat on each side five more times.

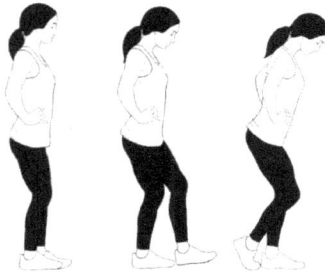

STRAIGHT-LINE WALKING

1. Stand next to a long wall, preferably a hallway.
2. Walk slowly making sure that the front foot's heel is touching the toe of the back foot. You can practice getting the position right over time.
3. Walk in this manner for at least 5 minutes.

If the wall is not long enough, you can always stop at the end and turn around.

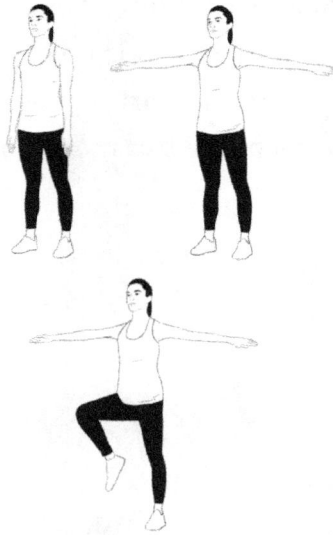

ROCKING THE BOAT

1. Stand up straight next to a wall or chair for support.
2. Keep your feet shoulder-width apart, and make sure you are balanced on your feet.
3. Slowly lift your arms to the side, keeping your head forward and your shoulders back.
4. As soon as you feel steady, slowly start to raise your right foot.
5. Bring your right knee as high as you can manage, and hold for 30 seconds.
6. Slowly lower your right foot.

7. Keep yourself steady, and slowly start to raise your left foot.
8. Bring your left knee as high as you can manage, and hold for 30 seconds.
9. Slowly lower your left foot.
10. Repeat on each side four more times.

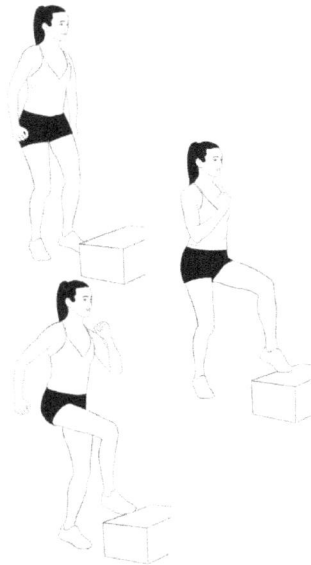

TAPPING FEET

1. Stand in front of a step—either an exercise step, a sturdy stool, or the bottom of a flight of stairs.
2. Make sure that there is something sturdy within reach should you need support.
3. Keep your feet apart at hip-width.

4. Lift your right leg up slowly, and tap the top of the step.

5. Lower your right foot down, and repeat 19 more times.

6. Lift your left leg up slowly, and tap the top of the step.

7. Lower your left foot down, and repeat 19 more times.

As you start feeling more balanced, you can step up onto the platform with each movement.

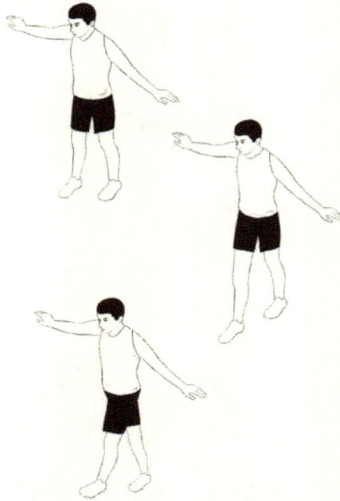

IMAGINARY TIGHTROPE WALKING

1. Stand next to a wall or chair.

2. Lift both your arms out to the sides.
3. Look at something ahead of you—an object in the distance—for focus.
4. Start to walk forward slowly, pausing for two to three seconds each time you raise each foot. 5. Take as many steps as you can but try to aim for at least 20 to 30.

This is good for posture and core strength training

CONCLUSION

Now that you know about all the benefits you can get from exercise—from mental to physical—it is clear that exercise will not just help you improve your mobility but also your life.

You also know why consistency is important to creating good habits and sticking to them, and you are equipped with some tips for staying on track.

I've explained what balance is and why it is important, as well as why we lose this ability as we get older. You know why falling is a risk as we get older, and also, how this doesn't have to mean a loss of freedom or health, as long as you exercise regularly.

Lastly, I have provided you with exercises from beginner to advanced so that you can start at your own pace and with support as needed. In time, as you grow stronger—and you will—you have exercises to continue with, as you embrace a healthy journey and lifestyle.

Remember, we can't help but get older but that doesn't mean that life has to get any less bright. You can gain back your independence and be stronger and fitter to enjoy life to the fullest. Just stay consistent.

REFERENCES

Avoiding a fall | Elderly fall prevention. (2020, December 15). *Age UK.* Www.ageuk.org.uk. https://www.ageuk.org.uk/information-advice/health-wellbeing/exercise/falls-prevention/

Balance Rules! (n.d.). *Science World.* Retrieved October 7, 2022, from https://www.scienceworld.ca/resource/balance-rules/#:~:text=In%20science%2C%20we%20say%20that

Bedosky, L. (2022, April 22). *The Best Core Exercises for Seniors.* Get Healthy U | Chris Freytag. https://gethealthyu.com/best-core-exercises-for-seniors/

Bremner, L. (2022, April 1). *The Power Of Consistency.* Luke Bremner Fitness - Personal Trainer Edinburgh. https://yourpersonaltraineredinburgh.com/power-of-consistency/

REFERENCES

Core Exercises for Seniors. Lifeline. (n.d.). Retrieved October 8, 2022, from https://www.lifeline.ca/en/resources/core-exercises-for-seniors/

Exercise and immunity. (n.d.). *MedlinePlus Medical Encyclopedia.* Medlineplus.gov. Retrieved October 7, 2022, from https://medlineplus.gov/ency/article/007165.htm#:~:text=Exercise%20causes%20change%20in%20antibodies

Exercise and Seniors. (2022, May). Familydoctor.org. https://familydoctor.org/exercise-seniors/ *Facts About Falls.* (2021, August 6). CDC. Www.cdc.gov. https://www.cdc.gov/falls/facts.html

Falls Prevention - What you need to know! (2021, August 3). Exercise Right. https://exerciseright.com.au/falls-prevention/

5 Benefits of Exercise for Seniors and Aging Adults | The GreenFields. (2020, October 25). The GreenFields Continuing Care Community | Lancaster, NY. https://thegreenfields.org/5-benefits-exercise-seniors-aging-adults/#:~:text=Exercise%20is%20good%20for%20you

14 Exercises for Seniors to Improve Strength and Balance. (n.d.). Philips Lifeline. Retrieved October 8, 2022, from https://www.lifeline.ca/en/resources/14-exercises-for-seniors-to-improve-strength-and-balance/

J. Campbell, B. (2020, July). *Exercise and Bone Health - Ortho-Info - AAOS.* Www.orthoinfo.org. https://orthoinfo.aaos.org/

en/staying-healthy/exercise-and-bone-health/#:~:text=Be-cause%20bo ne%20is%20living%20tissue

Jacobson, C. (2021, January 20). *Reducing falls for older adults: How physical activity keeps you balanced*. Scope. https://scope blog.stanford.edu/2021/01/20/reducing-falls-for-older-adults-how-physical-activity keeps-you-balanced/

McIntyre, K. (2022, January 7). *5 balance exercises that can help prevent falls*. Lifemark. https://www.lifemark.ca/blog-post/5-balance-exercises-can-help-prevent-falls

Melone, L. (n.d.). *7 Dynamic Warm Ups*. Www.arthritis.org. Retrieved October 8, 2022, from https://www.arthritis.org/health-wellness/healthy-living/physical-activity/other-activi ties/7-dyna mic-warm-ups

Minnis, G. (2020a, March 10). *Seated and Standing Chair Exercises for Seniors*. Healthline. https://www.healthline.com/health/chair-exercises-for-seniors

Minnis, G. (2020b, May 11). *Balance Exercises for Seniors: 11 Moves to Try*. Healthline. https://www.healthline.com/health/exercise-fitness/balance-exercises-for-seniors

Physical Activity in Ageing and Falls. (n.d.). Physiopedia. Retrieved October 6, 2022, from https://www.physio-pedia.com/Physical_Activity_in_Ageing_and_Falls?utm_source=physiopedia &utm_medium=related_articles&utm_cam-paign=ongoing_internal

REFERENCES

Preventing Falls: Exercises for Strength and Balance | HealthLink BC. (2020, December 7). Www.healthlinkbc.ca.

https://www.healthlinkbc.ca/healthy-eating-physical-activ ity/age-and-stage/older-adults/preventi   ng-falls-exercises-strength-and

Robinson, L., Smith, M., & Segal, J. (2022, October 6). *Exercise and Fitness as You Age*. HelpGuide.org. HelpGuide.org.

https://www.helpguide.org/articles/healthy-living/exercise-and-fitness-as-you-age.htm

Scalena, M. (2021, May 19). *7 Benefits of Daily Seated Exercise*. Sunshine Centres for Seniors. https://sunshinecentres.com/7-benefits-of-daily-seated-exercise/#:~:text=Strengthen-ing%20your %20muscles%20with%20seated

S.R., V. (2022, August 8). *What to Know About Core Exercises for Seniors?*. WebMD. https://www.webmd.com/fitness-exer cise/what-to-know-about-core-exercises-for-seniors

Standing Exercises for Seniors: 4 Easy Moves to Do at Home. (2020, June 11). Iora Primary Care. https://ioraprimarycare. com/blog/standing-exercises-for-seniors/

10 Balance Exercises for Seniors That You Can Do at Home. (2020, July 17). Snug Safety. https://www.snugsafe.com/all-posts/balance-exercises-for-seniors

The #1 Reason You Need Consistent Exercise. (2018, June 12). OSR Physical Therapy. https://www.osrpt.com/2018/06/reason-you-need-consistent-exercise/

12 Best Elderly Balance Exercises For Seniors to Reduce the Risk of Falls. (2019) Eldergym Senior Fitness. https://eldergym.com/elderly-balance/

Vestibular_Exercises. (n.d.).University of Mississippi Medical Center. Retrieved October 1, 2022, from https://www.umc.edu/Healthcare/ENT/Patient-Handouts/Adult/Otology/Vestibular_Exercises.ht ml

Van Pelt, J. (n.d.). *Fall Prevention: Targeted Exercise Reduces Risk - Today's Geriatric Medicine.* Www.todaysgeriatricmedicine.-com. Retrieved October 7, 2022, from https://www.todaysgeriatricmedicine.com/archive/JA21p28.shtml

William, B. (2020, November 19). *Core Exercises For Seniors: Your Exercise Days Aren't Behind You.* BetterMe Blog. https://betterme.world/articles/core-exercises-for-seniors/

WALL PILATES FOR SENIORS

SIMPLE EXERCISES TO PERFORM AT HOME THAT
IMPROVE FLEXIBILITY, MOBILITY, POSTURE, AND
BALANCE WHILE PROMOTING HEALTHY MOVEMENT

FIT FOREVER

FIT FOREVER

INTRODUCTION

In the world we live in today, 30 is the new 20, 40 is the new 30, and 50 is the new 40. People are aging backward! But not in an unnatural way. According to Thompson (2023), fitness programs for older adults rank fourth in the worldwide survey of fitness because as people get older, they have a burning desire to maintain energy, health, and longevity.

The World Health Organization Research (2022) also stated that people worldwide are living longer. Even though a number of seniors are getting more active, there is still a part of the older population that are in poor health due to a lack of activity.

You are among the elite who are ready to age gracefully through exercise. You have picked up this book because you are ready to begin preserving and restoring your health in small and simple ways every day so that you are able to pursue the things that you value through to an older age.

This book will introduce you to wall Pilates and, in return, only requires that you remain committed to daily exercising. Just like Rome was not built in a day, your physical fitness results will not be an overnight success.

When you begin to exercise, you open yourself to a lifelong mental and physical challenge that will improve the quality of all areas of your life. There are many benefits of committing to a life of fitness that we will discuss before diving into wall Pilates.

RECLAIM YOUR VITALITY

To some people, old age is a barren land where nothing grows anymore. That is mental slavery because you have the power to make healthy changes to your life no matter what age you are.

Society wants to put older adults in a cage by setting unrealistic timelines and standards, sending messages that if we do not find our purpose by 30 years old, then we are doomed. Or messages such as beauty and vitality have a time limit.

Those are lies. You can find your purpose in the golden years and endeavor to live an active life filled with bursts of energy to pursue your hobbies, a new career move, and even enhance your sex life with your spouse.

Whatever you value, you must know that it requires physical strength and that you can maintain your health and longevity. There are a number of benefits to living an active lifestyle.

Mental Benefits of an Active Lifestyle

Better Sleep

Frequent exercising increases body temperature and has the ability to reduce the number of hours it takes to fall asleep. However, it is not medically advised to participate in vigorous exercise during the evening hours.

Wall Pilates, which we will look at in this book, incorporates a light form of restful exercises that can actually be done later in the evening. Therefore, you can try the beginner forms of Pilates in the evening.

Decreases Stress-Related Issues

Issues such as depression, anxiety, stress, and other mood disorders can be gradually decreased through physical activity. A study by Callow et al. (2020) emphasized that older adults who engaged in physical fitness were seen to have reduced stress because exercising releases the production of endorphins.

Endorphins are hormones that are produced by the pituitary gland in the brain and act as messengers that release positive feelings. As you exercise, blood circulation also increases, and endorphins are passed through various regions of the brain, including the amygdala, which is responsible for generating fear-based responses to stress and emotional pain. Thus, exercising will help you have more control over your negative emotions and process them healthier.

Sharpens Focus

Exercising also creates new brain cells through a process known as neurogenesis. These fresh brain cells strengthen the hippocampus, which is responsible for cognitive functioning, learning, and memory formation in the brain. According to Schoenfeld & Swanson (2021), neurogenesis continues throughout our adult life and can be greatly enhanced by frequent exercises. Thus, exercising can help you improve your memory and learn new skills faster, even as you get older.

Physical Benefits of an Active Lifestyle

Improved Mobility

Healthy movement in the body is important to living a pain-free life, and increased mobility will achieve just that. Mobility is the range of motion in your joints which improves body movements, flexibility, and posture.

Increases Bone Density

According to the World Health Organization (2022), seniors usually struggle with osteoporosis which can invite a host of other problems, such as back pain. Frequent exercising helps to build more bone tissues and prevent osteoporosis.

Improves Cardiovascular Strength

Heart health is important for overall body health. Having a healthy heart will reduce the risks of stroke, high cholesterol, and heart disease. Exercising increases blood circulation levels and intensifies the amount of work that your heart does and subsequently strengthens it.

Understanding the benefits of living an active lifestyle may give you enthusiasm. Still, before we begin, I beseech you to make a promise to yourself to commit to taking care of your physical strength, to avoid the health issues that come as we age, and to pursue the things that you value.

BEFORE YOU BEGIN

Please note that this is a self-published book. The fitness advice in this book has been gathered through personal research and provided as an information resource. Thus, it cannot be used for any treatment purposes. If you are struggling with severe back or joint pain and have a hard time completing daily tasks, please visit a doctor.

You are responsible for ensuring your safety and are advised to do your own research before incorporating wall Pilates into your workout routines. Remember to warm up before an exercise and cool down afterward. The warm-up stretches provided are also great for cooling down. Furthermore, for all the exercises in this book, you will need an exercise mat.

Sets and Reps

The exercises in each chapter have a number of repetitions (reps) you can use to direct your exercises. You can also incorporate sets, which are a series of repetitions. For example, if an exercise includes 15 reps, and you repeat it for two sets, you would have done that exercise 30 times.

Maintain a one to two-minute rest between sets so you can breathe and focus on proper form during the exercises.

Determining Your Fitness Level

It will be helpful to test your fitness level so you can determine what to work on on your fitness journey. Below is a simple test that you can use. Remember to always listen to your doctor and pay attention to your own body's signals as you exercise. If something feels too painful, then stop.

Standing From Floor Test

This movement will test your strength, flexibility, and balance.

Sit on the floor, cross your legs, and then stand back up. Do so with the minimum amount of support that you think you need from your arms. When you first begin, you have 10 points. If you use your hands for support, subtract 1 point. If you use your knee for support, subtract 1 point. If you put one hand on your knee or thigh for support, then subtract another point. If you use your forearm for support, then subtract another point.

For example, if while you sat down, you put one of your hands on one of your knees, you have to subtract 1 point. If, when standing up, you use your knees and your hands to support the come up, you will have to subtract 2 points.

If your score is between 0 - 4, your fitness level could be improved with the beginner exercises found in this book. If your score is between 5 - 8, your fitness level could be developed with the intermediate exercises in this book. If your score is 9 or 10, you can continue your fitness journey using the advanced exercises.

1

ALL ABOUT WALL PILATES

Pilates is a workout that Joseph Pilates designed in the 20th Century to improve posture, flexibility, and strength through controlled body movements. Pilates is usually executed with a machine called a reformer that helps to control the movements by creating resistance.

The reformer can be replaced with a wall, hence the term 'Wall' Pilates. Therefore, wall Pilates is a variation of Pilates that use the resistance of a wall to improve flexibility, posture, and strength.

THE FUNDAMENTALS OF WALL PILATES

BREATHING

Breathing deeply by inhaling into the lower abdomen and exhaling forcefully by engaging the pelvic floor during an exhale is the main component of Pilates. Joseph Pilates first called Pilates 'Contrology' and stated that "breathing is the first act of life and the last" (Nesta, 2023). Therefore, breathing correctly can help bring balance to the mind and body.

According to Joseph Pilates, focusing on the breath during movements could help the Pilates practitioner to engage more fully in the exercise and reap its benefits.

ANCHORING

Anchoring, also known as centering, is the act of bringing awareness to the core while exercising. Pilates focuses on core engagement. The core is the group of muscles around the abdomen, lower back, hips, and buttocks. Having a strong core helps the body function properly because it enhances balance and overall body strength. Engaging the core in Pilates helps make the movements stronger and more fluid.

CONCENTRATION

Both breathing and anchoring throughout a Pilates movement require the practitioner to be fully focused. This aspect of Pilates, therefore, increases mindfulness and helps the practitioner reap maximum benefits from the movement.

ALIGNMENT

Pilates requires precise movements and alignment with the whole body. Pilates is done with a correct posture of the spine and muscles so that the movements are fluid. The goal of alignment in Pilates is to fix any incorrect posturing in the practitioner that will benefit him even after the exercise.

IS WALL PILATES EFFECTIVE FOR SENIORS?

With a number of buzzing fitness centers to choose from, you may be skeptical about performing at-home exercises. However, wall Pilates is effective because the wall acts not only as a strengthening tool by providing resistance but also as a teacher to provide feedback and correct posture.

The wall will help you achieve good form, which is essential to an effective workout. Placing your feet, hands, and spine on the wall while executing Pilates will help you find alignment by listening to your body. Thus, you will be able to tweak your posture as though you have an instructor adjusting your movements.

Aside from bad posture, there are a number of maladies that we face when we begin to age. A few of these include:

- Hip and joint injuries
- Falling easily
- Multiple sclerosis
- Osteoporosis
- Labored breathing

IMPROVES SPINAL ALIGNMENT

The alignment principle in Pilates will challenge seniors to engage in movements that will straighten out the body's frame, thus preventing sclerosis and reducing its symptoms significantly.

IMPROVES CORE STRENGTH

Anchoring and focusing on the core while engaging in Pilates movement will challenge seniors to strengthen the muscles that improve balance, thus reducing the proclivity to falling easily. This core strength will help alleviate hip and joint pains because the body will be strong enough to carry its own weight.

IMPROVES FLEXIBILITY AND MOBILITY

Pilates is a combination of strength training and flexibility training simultaneously. Continuously lengthening and strengthening the muscles will increase seniors' mobility and flexibility.

IMPROVES OVERALL WELL-BEING

Focused breathing will increase mindfulness for seniors and reduce labored breathing. The amount of concentration it takes to integrate all the fundamentals of Pilates in a workout will help alleviate a lot of problems. Pilates can increase bone density which may prevent osteoporosis in seniors.

Try the Pilates in the following chapters and begin reaping the benefits.

2

BEGINNER WALL PILATES

The Pilates in this section are great for beginners. You do not have to do it all in one workout session. If you scored zero points or one point on the fitness test, choose three exercises and do two sets. If you scored three or four points, you could start with five movements for two sets and build strength from there. Ensure to do all the warm-ups.

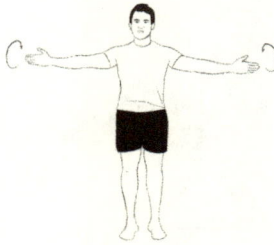

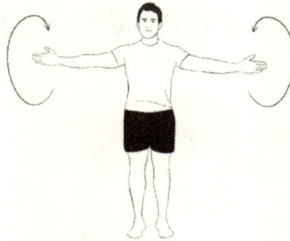

ARM ROLLS

1. Raise your arms sideways.
2. Make small circles in the air 10 times in a clockwise direction, then counterclockwise.
3. After that, make bigger circles in both clockwise and counterclockwise directions.
4. Do those 10 times as well.

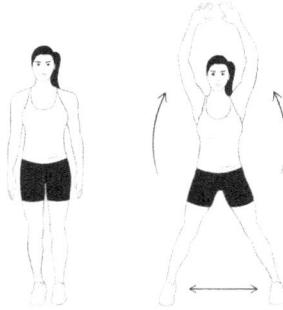

JUMPING JACKS

1. Stand with your legs together and your arms at your sides.
2. Then, jump out to a hip-width position, and as you jump, extend your arms over your head.
3. Jump back into the starting position.
4. Repeat these 15 more times.

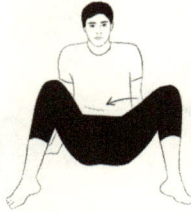

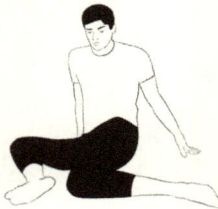

HIP ROTATIONS

1. Sit down on your mat and support yourself by putting your arms behind you on the ground.
2. Lift your legs to make an A shape between the ground and your legs.
3. Drop both your legs slowly to the left side and let your head follow to the left as well.
4. Repeat this 10 times.
5. Repeat steps 1 - 4 on the right side.

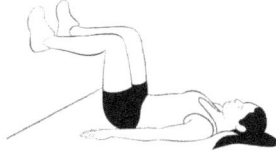

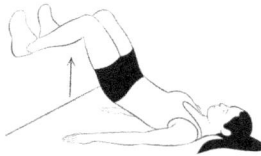

WALL GLUTE BRIDGES

1. Lie down on the mat with your legs facing the wall.
2. Firmly place your feet on the wall, ensuring that your legs are hip-width apart and maintaining a 90-degree angle to the floor.
3. Then, squeeze your glutes and raise your pelvis off the ground. Maintain a tight core while doing this exercise.
4. Hold this position for 60 seconds, making sure that you are breathing throughout.
5. Drop your pelvis.
6. Repeat this 10 times.

WALL SQUATS

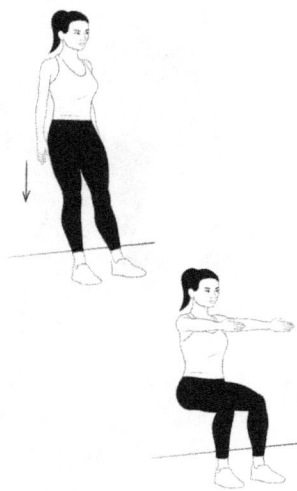

1. Stand with your back pressed on the wall.
2. Place your feet hip-width apart.
3. Tuck in your pelvis and lift your arms forward in front of you.
4. Bend your knees and slowly drop into a seated position until your thighs are parallel to the floor (90 degrees). Inhale as you bend down.
5. Hold for 30 seconds.
6. Slowly stand back up, and as you do, put your arms back to your side. Exhale as you stand up.
7. Repeat this 5 times.

WALL CRUNCHES

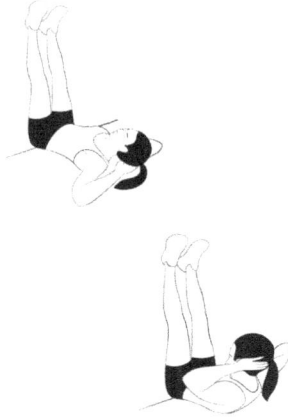

1. Lie down on your back on your mat.
2. Place your feet on the wall as if doing the wall bridge exercise above.
3. Place your hands behind your head.
4. With your eyes facing the ceiling, inhale, then lift your shoulders off the ground as you exhale.
5. Slowly come back down to the starting position as you inhale.
6. Repeat this 10 times.

STANDING ARM MOVEMENTS

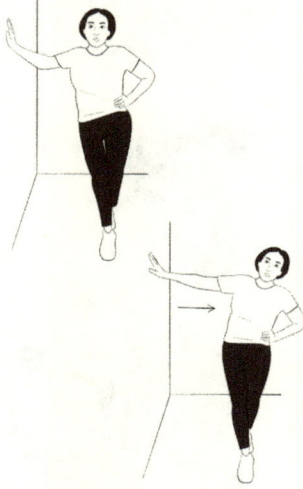

1. Stand with your right side facing the wall and place your hand on the wall.
2. Place your left foot in front of your right foot as if you were getting ready to run.
3. Place your left hand on your left hip.
4. Bend your arm towards the wall while you inhale.
5. Bend your arm away from the wall while you exhale.
6. Repeat this 15 times on the right side and 15 times on the left side.

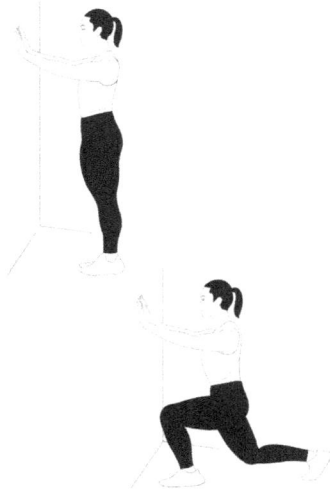

FORWARD LUNGES

1. While standing, face the wall and place your arms on the wall.
2. Step back with your feet, so your starting position resembles a diagonal line.
3. Next, step forward with your right leg and bend it, so your right thigh is parallel to the ground.
4. Step back and repeat the move on the right leg 15 times.
5. Then repeat the move on the left leg.

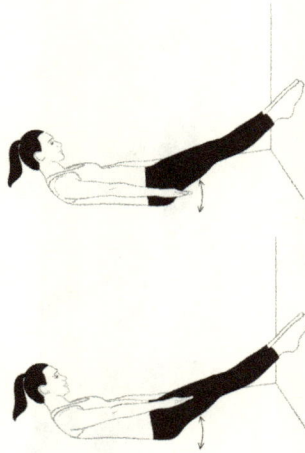

HUNDREDS

1. Lie down on your mat.
2. And place your feet diagonally on the wall.
3. Straighten your arms at your side and lift them off the mat.
4. Pump your arms up and down while taking deep breaths (breathe into the count of four and breathe out to the count of four).
5. Repeat this for 10 breaths (one inhale and one exhale equals one full breath).

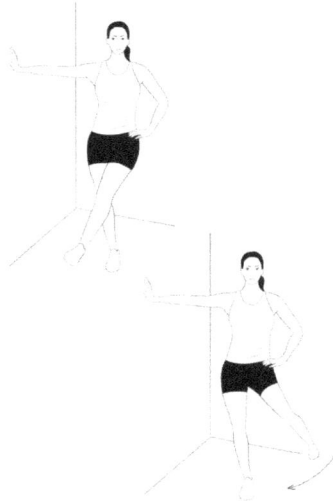

SIDE LEG SWING

1. Stand sideways towards a wall with your right hand firmly placed on the wall.
2. Step away from the wall so that your arm is extended, but do not move your hand away.
3. Next, lift your left leg, swing it forward across your right leg, and then swing it backward. Inhale as you swing it forward, and exhale as you swing it backward.
4. Repeat this motion 10 times.
5. Repeat steps 3 and 4 on the right leg.

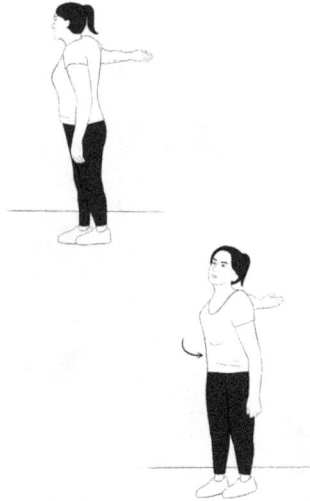

CHEST OPENERS

1. Stand sideways facing a wall, extend your right arm backward, and place your hand on the wall. Ensure that your head is facing straight at all times and your hand is parallel with the floor.
2. Slowly rotate your torso to the left side while inhaling. Keep your head up, and do not tuck it in.
3. Hold step two for 15 seconds.
4. Then, slowly rotate back to the starting position while exhaling.
5. Repeat this motion 10 times.
6. Repeat steps 2 - 5 with your left arm placed on the wall.

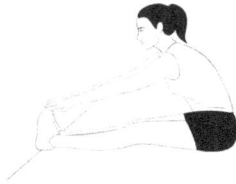

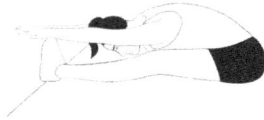

SEATED FORWARD ROLL

1. Sit down on your mat facing the wall. Ensure your core is engaged and sit tall (do not slump your shoulders forward).
2. Make sure your feet are touching the wall and stretch your arms out in front of you.
3. Draw your navel into your spine and lower your back to the ground slowly as far as you can go while exhaling. Keep your navel sucked in towards your spine the whole time.
4. Then, take a deep breath and lean your torso forward until your hands touch the wall (if only your fingertips touch the wall or you only reach halfway, that is okay, do not push your flexibility levels too

quickly). Keep your arms parallel to the floor for the entire motion.

5. Repeat this 10 times.

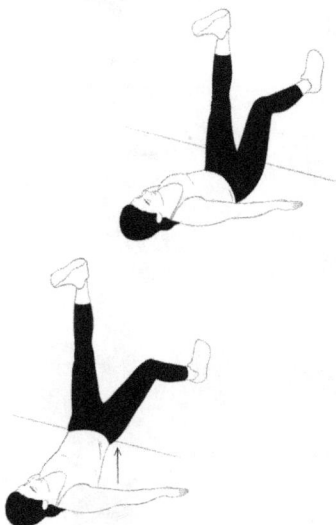

SINGLE LEG BRIDGES

1. Lie down on your mat and place your feet on the wall, ensuring they are at a 90-degree angle.
2. Lift your right leg in the air and flex your toes.
3. Then, lift your pelvis slowly while inhaling.
4. Bring your pelvis down to the ground slowly while exhaling.
5. Repeat 10 times on each leg.

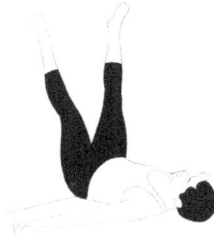

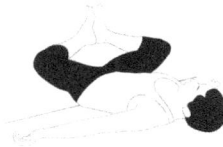

WALL-ASSISTED BUTTERFLY

1. Lie down with your back on your mat with your rear end pressed on the wall.
2. Ensure that your navel is pressed inwards, so there is no gap between the mat and your back.
3. Next, lift your legs and open them to make a V shape on the wall.
4. Then, bring the soles of your feet inwards until they touch. If you feel flexible enough or are ready to challenge yourself, lower your legs in this butterfly position until they are closer to your rear end but still on the wall.
5. Finally, close your knees while exhaling and open them again while inhaling.

6. Each time you open and close your legs in the butterfly position is a count of one. Repeat for a count of 10.

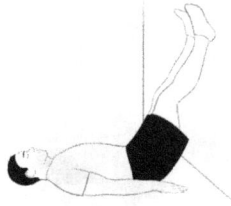

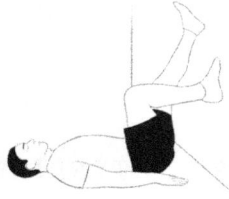

KNEE BENDS

1. Lie down on your back with your arms relaxed on the mat beside you.
2. Relax your neck, open your chest, and ensure your spine is in a neutral position so that there is no arch forming between your back and the mat.
3. Place your feet on the wall in a 90-degree position.
4. Breathe deeply and engage your pelvic floor muscles. Your stomach will feel tight when your pelvic floor is engaged.

5. Inhale and bend your right knee towards you. Keep your leg in a 90-degree position when it is off the wall.
6. Hold for three seconds while keeping your abdominal muscles and pelvic floor engaged.
7. Put your leg back on the wall.
8. Repeat this 10 times on each leg.

STANDING LEG CURLS

1. Stand facing a wall and extend your arms outwards until your hands are firmly planted on the wall.
2. Lean your body forward, engage your pelvis and abdominal muscles, and maintain this position.
3. Next, slowly lift the soles of your left foot until you almost touch your hind leg.
4. Put your left foot back down slowly and repeat with the right foot.
5. Do this 10 times on each side.

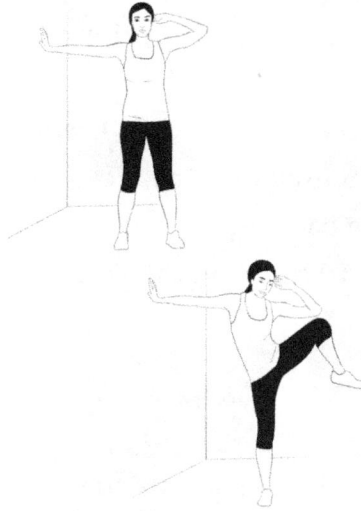

STANDING CRUNCHES

1. Stand with your right side facing the wall and extend your arm to your side until your hand is firmly planted on the wall.
2. Place your feet hip-width apart.
3. Raise your left arm slowly to the ceiling.
4. Crunch your left elbow down as you raise your left knee. Your elbow and knee should touch, then extend your arm up again and place your leg down. Remember to inhale as you extend upwards and exhale as you crunch.
5. Repeat this motion on your left side 10 times and again on the right side 10 more times.

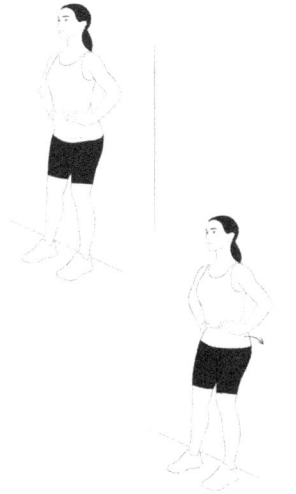

WALL-ASSISTED PELVIC TILT

1. Stand with your back against the wall.
2. Place your feet hip-width apart.
3. Place your hands on your feet.
4. Contract your abdominal muscles and tilt your pelvis forward. When you tilt, there should be no gap between your lower back and the wall.
5. Tilt the pelvis backward again.
6. Repeat this motion 10 times.

3

INTERMEDIATE WALL PILATES

Attempt these movements only when you are able to complete all the beginner movements twice without intense strain. If you scored five or six points on the fitness test, then choose five exercises for two sets. If you scored seven or eight points, attempt six exercises for two sets. Remember to do all the warm-ups.

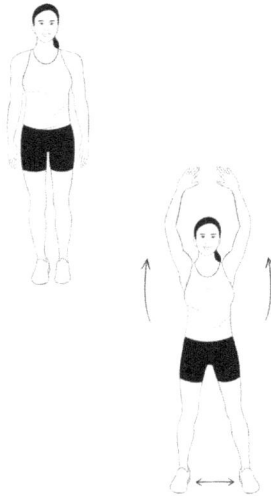

JUMPING JACKS

1. Stand with your legs together and your arms at your sides.
2. Then, jump out to a hip-width position, and as you jump, extend your arms over your head.
3. Jump back into the starting position.
4. Repeat these 20 more times.

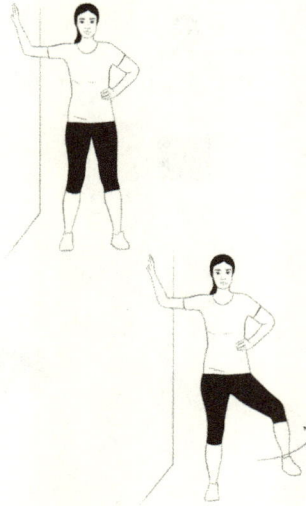

HIP CIRCLES

1. Stand with your arm against a wall.
2. Raise your left leg up and rotate it outwards.
3. Repeat this motion 15 times.
4. Then turn your left leg inwards.
5. Repeat this motion 15 times.
6. Drop your left leg and do the same on the right leg.

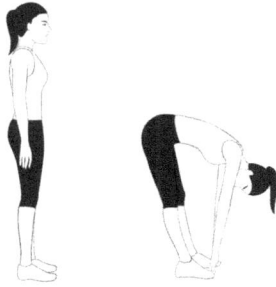

TOE TOUCHES

1. Stand straight with your legs together.
2. Next, bend down, loosening your back and letting your head relax, and reach your arms as far as you can go. If you can touch your toes, great; if you cannot, that is okay.
3. Come up very slowly, and lift your spine one vertebra at a time, roll your shoulders, lift your neck, and then lift your head and roll it back.
4. Do this five times.

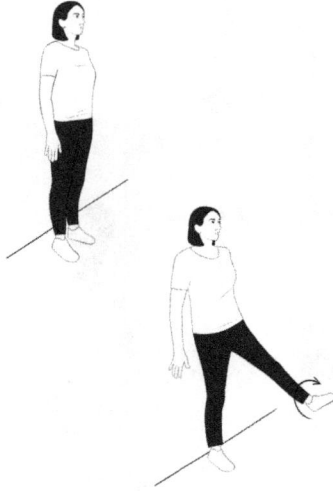

SINGLE LEG CIRCLES

1. Stand tall with your back against the wall.
2. Engage your abdominal muscles and tilt your pelvis, so there is no arch in your back or gap between your lower back and the wall.
3. Next, lift your leg off the ground and rotate it to the left 20 times.
4. Rotate it to the right 15 times.
5. Drop your left leg and repeat on the right leg.

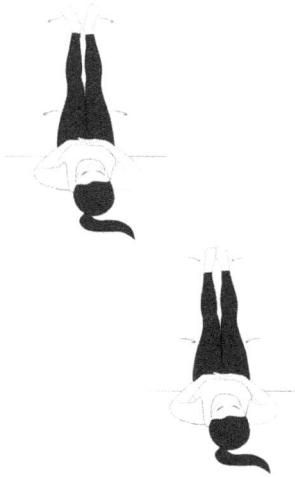

WALL INVERSION

1. Lie down on your mat and raise your legs up on the wall.
2. Rotate your thighs inwards, so your toes touch each other.
3. Rotate your thighs outwards, so your toes are facing outward.
4. Repeat this motion for a count of 15.

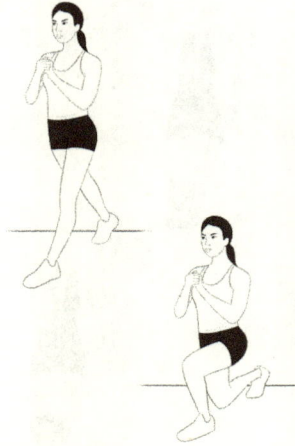

LUNGE SQUAT

1. Stand a short distance away from the wall with your back facing the wall.
2. Place your left foot on the wall with only the sole of your foot touching the wall.
3. Engage your abdominal muscles and bend down until your right thigh is parallel to the ground.
4. Repeat this 15 times on both legs.

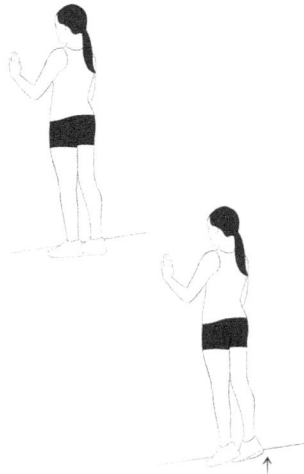

CALF RAISES

1. Stand facing the wall.
2. Lengthen your arms and fix your hands on the wall.
3. Bend forward with your whole body, tuck your pelvis inwards, and maintain that position.
4. Slowly raise the heels of both feet while inhaling until you are standing on the ball of your feet.
5. Slowly drop your feet while exhaling.
6. Repeat 15 times.

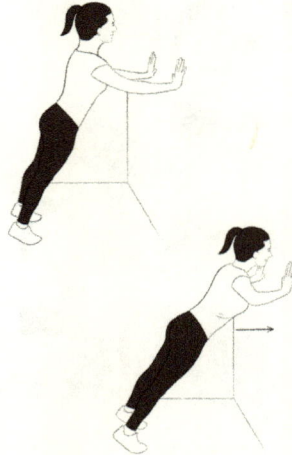

WALL-ASSISTED PUSH-UPS

1. Stand facing the wall.
2. Lengthen your arms and fix your hands on the wall.
3. Bend forward with your whole body, tuck your pelvis inwards, and maintain that position.
4. Pull away from the wall.
5. Repeat the motion 15 times while breathing.

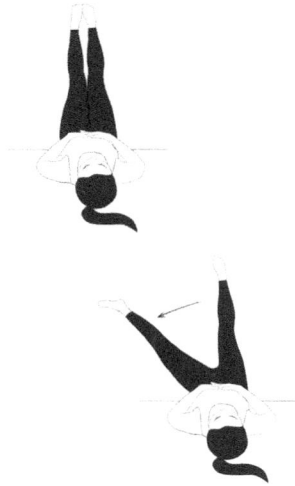

HIP OPENERS

1. Lie down on your mat and place your feet on the wall.
2. Slightly tilt your pelvis forward as you tighten your abdomen to ensure there is no space between the mat and your spine.
3. Next, pull your left leg slightly off the wall and point your toes.
4. Then, open your left leg sideways until you touch the ground with it or as far as you can.
5. Finally, bring it back up to the starting position.
6. Repeat this 15 times on each leg.

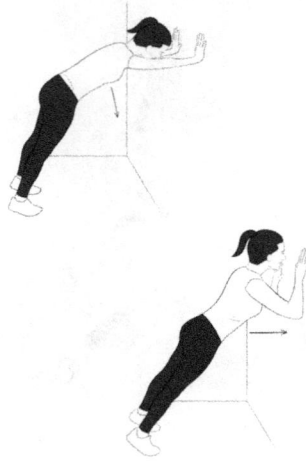

PIKES AND PLANKS

1. Stand facing the wall.
2. Lengthen your arms and fix your hands on the wall.
3. Bend down while engaging your abdomen until your torso is parallel to the floor. This is a pike.
4. Come back up and immediately lean your whole body forward into a wall plank.
5. One pike and one plank together make a count of one. Repeat this 15 times.

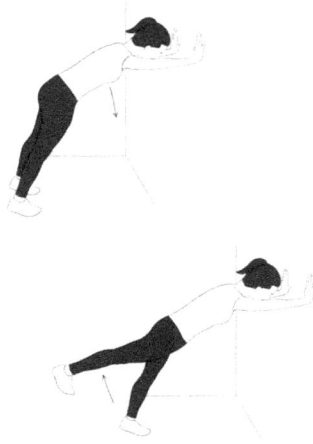

LEG LIFTS

1. Stand facing the wall and extend your arms to touch the wall.
2. Lean forward until your torso is aligned with the ground.
3. Tighten your abdominal muscles and extend your left leg back without arching your back.
4. Slowly bring it back down but do not touch the mat and raise it again.
5. Repeat this 15 times on both legs.

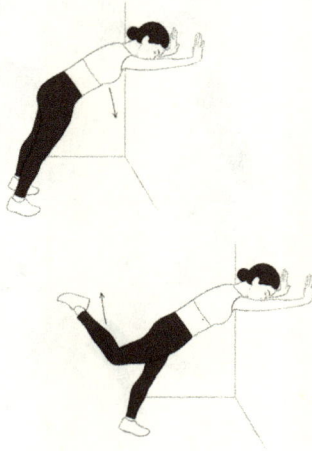

DONKEY KICKS

1. Stand facing the wall and extend your arms to touch the wall.
2. Lean forward until your torso is aligned with the ground.
3. Tighten your abdominal muscles and bend forward until your body is parallel to the floor.
4. Raise your right leg to make a V-shape with your leg without arching your back.
5. With your toes pointed, kick the right leg up and down.
6. Repeat this 15 times on both legs.

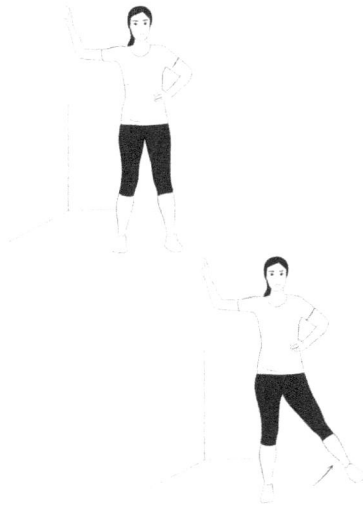

SIDE LEG LIFTS

1. Stand sideways with the wall and place your right arm on the wall at a 90-degree angle.
2. Lean sideways to support your body with the wall.
3. Then, slowly lift your leg to the side as high as you can and bring it back down.
4. Repeat this 15 times on both legs.

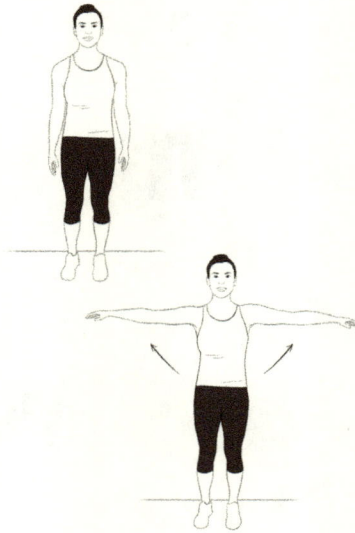

STANDING ARM RAISES

1. With your back against the wall, place your feet 2 inches apart.
2. Tuck your pelvis inwards, ensuring there is no space between your lower back and the wall.
3. Tighten your abdominal muscles and slowly raise your arms until they are parallel to the floor.
4. Hold for four deep breaths and slowly lower your arms back to your side.
5. Repeat 15 times.

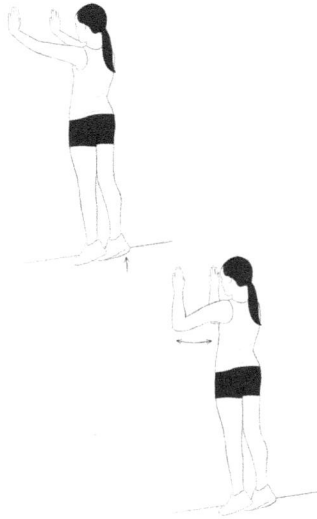

TRICEP DIPS

1. Extend your arms towards the wall and place your hands firmly on the wall.
2. Walk your hands up the wall until they are at the same height as your forehead.
3. Lift your heels and stand only on the ball of your feet.
4. Then, bend your elbows as low as you can and then extend your arms out again.
5. Repeat this 15 times.

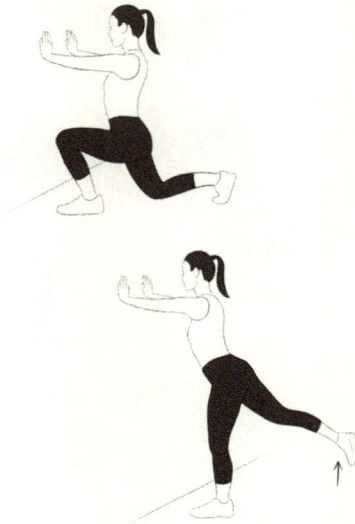

LUNGE TO KICKBACKS

1. Stand with your arms extended towards the wall.
2. While holding the wall, take a step back with your left leg.
3. Bend down until your right thigh is parallel to the floor.
4. Slowly lift yourself back up and immediately kick your left leg up as high as you can.
5. Do this 15 times on both legs.

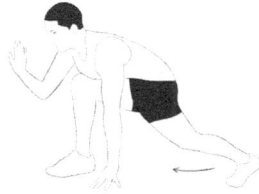

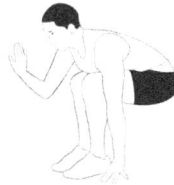

RUNNER'S LUNGES

1. Stand sideways with your right hand placed on the wall.
2. Engage your core, and step back with your left foot.
3. As you do that, touch the ground with the fingertips of your left hand. (It should look like you are about to start running).
4. Lift your left leg forward and ensure it is parallel to the floor.
5. Repeat this 15 times on both legs.

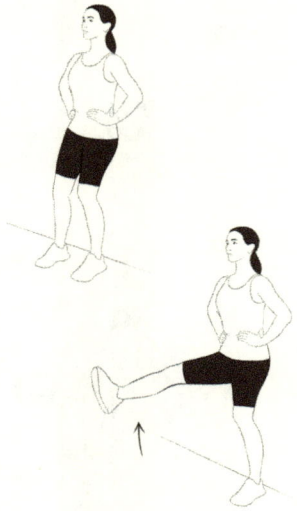

MARCHING LIFT ON WALL

1. Stand with your back against the wall and bend your legs slightly.
2. Slightly move your legs forward.
3. After that, tighten your abdomen and tilt your pelvis, so there is no space between your lower spine and the wall.
4. Then, slowly lift one leg at a time and aim to maintain a straight back. Do not rock sideways.
5. Repeat this for 15 counts.

4

ADVANCED WALL PILATES

O nly attempt these movements when you can do all the intermediate Pilates movements for one set without straining. If you scored nine points on the fitness test, choose six movements. If you scored ten points, start with ten movements for one set.

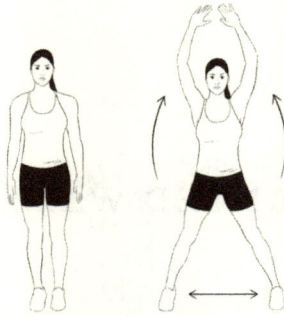

JUMPING JACKS

1. Start with your legs together and your arms at your sides.
2. Then, jump out to a hip-width position, and as you jump, extend your arms over your head.
3. Jump back into the starting position.
4. Repeat these 20 more times.

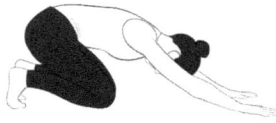

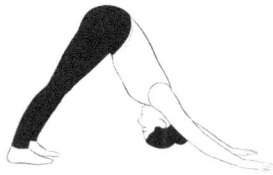

DOWNWARD DOG

1. Kneel down on all fours.
2. Then, lift your knees off the ground while simultaneously extending your arms.
3. Your body should make a V-shape.
4. Hold this pose for 15 seconds and slowly bring your knees forward and arms back to the starting position.

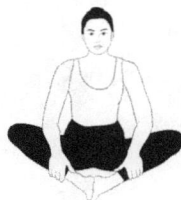

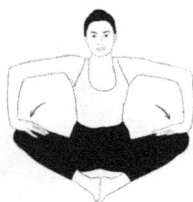

BUTTERFLY STRETCH

1. Sit down with your legs folded into a diamond shape. Your feet should be touching.
2. Sit up tall.
3. Then, push your knees outward as far as you can go.
4. Hold for 20 seconds and repeat it twice.

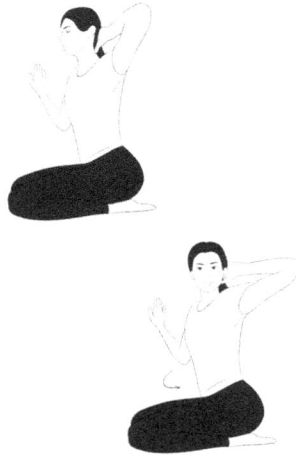

SIDE CRUNCHES

1. Kneel on your mat and straighten your torso.
2. Place one arm on the wall and place another behind your head.
3. Crunch to the side as you exhale, then come back up as you inhale.
4. Repeat 20 times on each side.

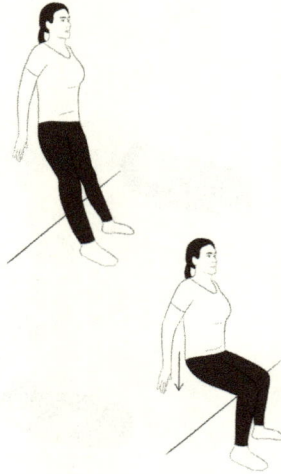

ROLL DOWN

1. Stand with your back against the wall.
2. Next, move your feet forward about 2m away from the wall.
3. Pull your abdominal muscles in and keep your arms at your sides.
4. Tuck your chin on your chest and begin to roll your back down slowly while inhaling. One vertebra at a time.
5. Roll down as far as you can go, keeping your abdomen engaged and keeping your hips against the wall.

6. Begin to exhale and roll your spine back up one vertebra at a time until you are standing tall against the wall again.
7. Repeat this 15 times.

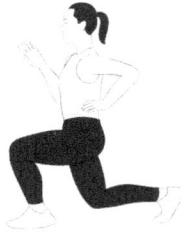

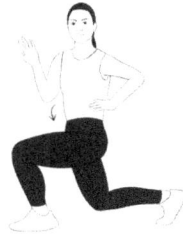

LUNGE TWIST

1. Stand sideways with the wall and place your hand on the wall.
2. After that, step forward with your leg while standing tall. Straighten out your spine like there is a rope pulling you up from the center of your head.
3. Bend down until your thighs are parallel to the floor.
4. Next, twist your torso sideways, then back to the front.

5. Stand up and step backward.
6. Do it again on the other leg.
7. Repeat this 20 times.

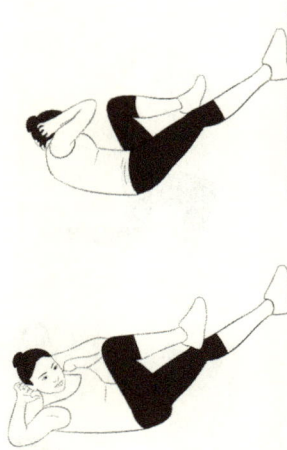

CRUNCH PULSES

1. Lie on your mat and place your legs high up on the wall.
2. Place your hands behind your head.
3. Engage your core and ensure that there is no space between the mat and your spine.
4. After that, bend your right knee and lift your left shoulder off the ground, so your left elbow touches the right knee.
5. Pulse 15 times in this position while breathing.

6. Bring your shoulder back down.
7. Repeat on the other side.

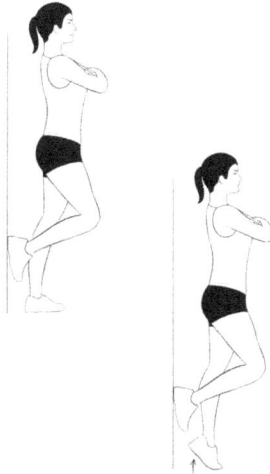

ONE-LEG CALF RAISES

1. Stand with your back facing the wall and place your right foot on the wall for balance.
2. After that, fold your arms out in front of you.
3. Then, raise your left leg slowly until you are standing only on the ball of your foot.
4. Then, slowly come back down to your heels.
5. Repeat this 20 times on both legs.

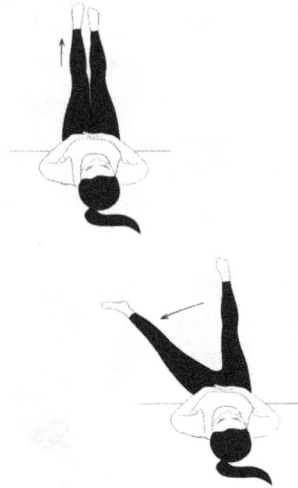

EXTENDED HIP OPENERS

1. Lie down on your mat and place your feet on the wall.
2. Slightly tilt your pelvis forward as you tighten your abdomen to ensure there is no space between the mat and your spine.
3. After that, lift your right leg as high as you can go without bending the knee.
4. Then, drop it down slowly to the side as far as you can go, ensuring that your core is engaged the whole time.
5. Bring it back up in the air.
6. Repeat this motion 20 times on both legs.

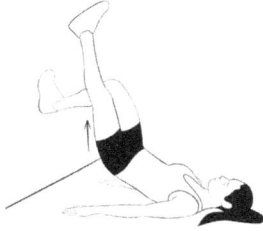

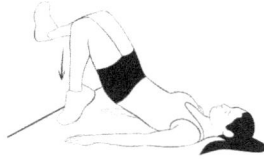

GLUTE BRIDGE WITH TOE TAP

1. Get into a glute position as though you are about to do a wall glute bridge.
2. Raise your hips off the ground.
3. While your hips are off the ground, lift your left leg up and then tap your toe on the ground.
4. Place your left leg back on the wall and drop your hips slowly to the ground.
5. Repeat this motion on the left side 15 times and then on the right leg 15 times.

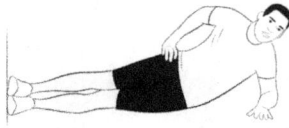

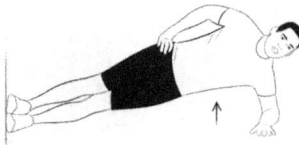

SIDE PLANKS

1. Lie down on your mat with your right side.
2. Place your right arm at a 90-degree angle, as it will be your main support.
3. Plant your feet on the wall, having the left leg 2 inches above the right leg.
4. Bend both legs slightly.
5. Next, put your left arm on the mat in front of you for support.
6. Then, straighten your legs and lift yourself off the ground slowly.
7. Slowly come back down.
8. Repeat this 20 times, resting when you need to.

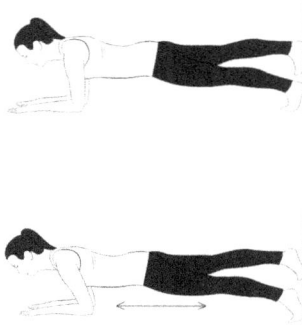

DOLPHIN PLANKS

1. Lie down on your mat with your face away from the way.
2. Place your forearms at a 90-degree angle and plant your feet on the wall.
3. Lift yourself up and then move your left leg 2 inches above the right leg.
4. Tighten your abdominal muscles and tilt your pelvis inwards.
5. After that, push yourself forward until only the balls of your feet are on the wall.
6. Next, push yourself backward.
7. Keep moving back and forth, keeping your core engaged for 10 breaths.

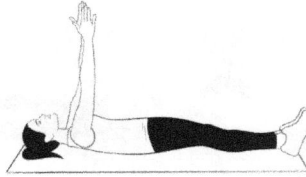

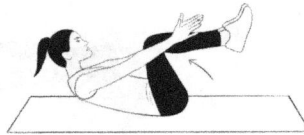

TABLETOP CRUNCHES

1. Lie down on your mat and place your feet against the wall, ensuring your thighs are parallel to the floor.
2. Extend both arms all the way over your head and keep them straight.
3. Engage your abdominal muscles, so there is no space between your lower back and the floor.
4. After that, pull your knees towards you as you slightly lift your shoulders off the ground and extend your arms towards your legs (Crunch).
5. Then, release the crunch and go back to the starting position.
6. Remember to breathe through the movements.
7. Repeat this crunching movement 15 times.

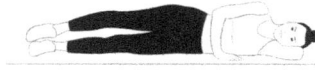

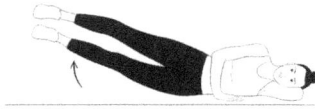

LYING SIDE LEG LIFTS

1. Lie down on your right side on the mat with your whole body leaning against the wall.
2. Extend your right arm forward on the floor for balance.
3. Engage your core.
4. Then, lift both your legs upwards, with your heels always touching the wall.
5. After that, bring them back down.
6. Repeat this motion for 15 breaths.

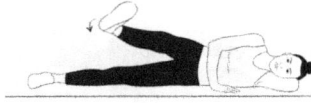

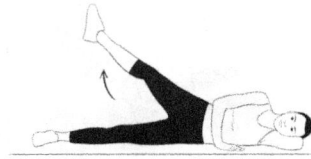

LYING SINGLE-LEG LIFT

1. Lie down on your right side on the mat with your whole body leaning against the wall.
2. Place your right forearm on the floor for balance.
3. Engage your core.
4. Move your right leg forward and lift it up, then down.
5. Repeat this 10 times on each leg.

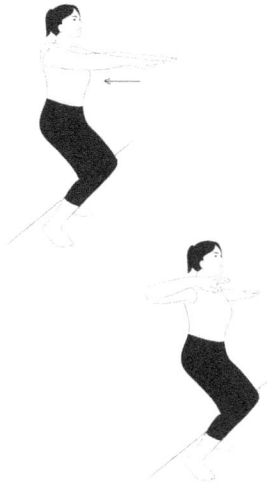

ARM EXERCISES

1. Stand with your back against the wall.
2. Tilt your pelvis, so there is no space between your spine and the wall.
3. Bend down slightly, or if you can, bend into a full wall squat.
4. Then, extend your arms forward in front of you and pull them toward the wall at a 90-degree angle.
5. Repeat this motion for 10 counts.

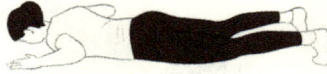

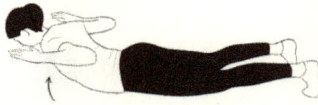

BACK EXTENSIONS

1. Lie with your face down on your mat.
2. Press your feet against the wall.
3. Bring your arms forward, placing your hands right in front of your forehead.
4. Squeeze your glutes and lift your chest off the ground as you exhale.
5. Hold for three seconds and come back down.
6. Repeat this movement 10 times.

CONCLUSION

With all the exercises in this book, reclaiming your vitality will be easier for you. One downfall you need to be aware of is the all-or-nothing mentality. Believing that you must never miss a day of exercising will only deter your progress.

Just because you fall off for one day or one week does not mean you need to restart your fitness journey or give up. Simply pick up from where you left off and keep progressing.

Here are a few ways you can become consistent rather than perfect.

1. Set schedules that work with your lifestyle.
2. Maintain a weekly routine.
3. Set realistic goals.

4. Monitor your progress.
5. Have rest days.
6. Reward yourself.

Remember, you can have the energy to spend time with your loved ones, be independent, and pursue your passions. All it takes from you is consistency.

REFERENCES

Bubb, F. (2016, October 8). *7 Great Benefits of Pilates for Seniors*. Elite Therapy. http://elite-therapy.com/7-great-bene fits-of-pilates-for-seniors/

Bushman, L. (2023). *Beginner Full Body Pilates on the Wall*. YouTube. https://www.youtube.com/watch?v= _VIu33oxs_I&list=TLPQMDMwMzIwMjNjk0hbuN VR_w&index=6

Callow, D. D., Arnold-Nedimala, N. A., Jordon, L. S., Pena, G. S., Won, J., Woodard, J. L., & Smith, J. C. (2020, October). The Mental Health Benefits of Physical Activity in Older Adults Survive the COVID-19 Pandemic. *The American Journal of Geriatric Psychiatry, 28*(10), 1046-1057. https://doi.org/10. 1016/j.jagp.2020.06.024

Cleveland Clinic. (2022, May 19). *Endorphins: What they are and how to boost them?* Cleveland Clinic. https://my.cleveland clinic.org/health/body/23040-endorphins#:~:text=Endor-phins%20are%20created%20in%20your

Foundation Chiropractic. (n.d.). *At Home Fitness Testing.* https://foundationchiropractic.ca/at-home-fitness-testing/

Herman, E. (2022). *Pilates For Dummies.* Wiley. https://books.google.com.my/books?hl=en&lr=&id=GF-LEAAAQBAJ&oi=fnd&pg=PA3&dq=wall+pilates&ots=TD8O55aLhG&sig=2YsLd6I38ZiTe_eEempK6tiotZw&redir_esc=y#v=onepage&q=wall%20pilates&f=false

Hutchens, F. (2021, January 5). *Are You As Fit As You Could Be For Your Age? Find Out By Taking 4 Fitness Tests — Movementum.* Movementum. https://movementum.co.uk/journal/fitness-tests

LaMeaux, E. C. (2023). *8 Principles of Pilates.* Gaiam. https://www.gaiam.com/blogs/discover/8-principles-of-pilates

Larbi, M. (2023, February 22). *Wall pilates is the new low-impact exercise everyone's trying – but is it worth your time?* Stylist. https://www.stylist.co.uk/fitness-health/workouts/wall-pilates-low-impact-benefits/745307

Mayo Clinic. (2019). *5 steps to start a fitness program.* Mayo Clinic. https://www.mayoclinic.org/healthy-lifestyle/fitness/in-depth/fitness/art-20048269

Mayo Clinic. (2021, October 8). *7 great reasons why exercise matters.* https://www.mayoclinic.org/healthy-lifestyle/ fitness/in-depth/exercise/art-20048389#:~:text=Exer-cise%20boosts%20energy&text=Regular%20physical%20ac-tivity%20can%20improve

McGuire, J. (2023, January 19). *Wall Pilates is the new workout everyone is talking about — here's what happened when I tried it.* Tom's Guide. https://www.tomsguide.com/news/wall-pilates-is-the-new-workout-everyone-is-talking-about-heres-what-happened-when-i-tried-it

Mukhwana, J., & Munuhe, N. (2022, November 9). *Wall Pilates Guide For The Beginner Looking For A Sculpted Body.* BetterMe. https://betterme.world/articles/wall-pilates/

NESTA. (2020, December 3). *The 10 Guiding Principles of Pilates | What is Pilates?* https://www.nestacertified.com/the-10-principles-of-pilates/

Ogle, M. (2021, May 21). *6 Pilates Principles to Integrate Mind, Body, and Spirit.* Verywell Fit. https://www.verywellfit.com/ six-pilates-principles-2704854

Pilates on Demand. (2023). *Pilates Single Leg Circle on the Wall.* YouTube. https://www.youtube.com/watch?v= KHO80OHfoZQ&t=8s

Prvulovic, T. (2022, January 14). *How Fit Should You Be at 60? - 5 Key Fitness Tests for Older Adults.* Second Wind Movement.

https://secondwindmovement.com/how-fit-should-you-be-at-60/

Schoenfeld, T. J., & Swanson, C. (2021, July 21). A Runner's High for New Neurons? Potential Role for Endorphins in Exercise Effects on Adult Neurogenesis. *Biomolecules, 11*(8), 1077. https://doi.org/10.3390/biom11081077

Shea, N. (2023, February 10). *Wall Pilates Guide for Beginners | MYPROTEIN™*. Myprotein. https://www.myprotein.com/thezone/training/wall-pilates-guide-for-beginners/

Thompson, W. R. (2023). Worldwide Survey of Fitness Trends for 2023. *ACSM's Health & Fitness Journal, 27*(1), 9-18. https://doi.org/10.1249/FIT.0000000000000834

Tipane, J., Sullivan, C., & Ajmera, R. (2021, April 22). *19 Pilates Benefits Backed By Science*. Healthline. https://www.healthline.com/nutrition/pilates-benefits#what-it-is

Trifecta Pilates. (2023). *Pilates Wall Workout | 40 Min Full Body Pilates*. YouTube. https://www.youtube.com/watch?v=fQDb3rbfTkg&list=TLPQMDMwMzIwMjNjk0hbuNVR_w&index=7

World Health Organization (WHO). (2022, October 1). *Ageing and health*. https://www.who.int/news-room/fact-sheets/detail/ageing-and-health

www.ingramcontent.com/pod-product-compliance
Lightning Source LLC
Chambersburg PA
CBHW031123020426
42333CB00012B/202